ECG / EKG INTERPRETATION

A Systematic Approach to read a 12-lead ECG and interpreting Heart Rhythms in 15 Seconds or Less without Memorization

Dr. Gabriel J. Connor

CONTENTS

PORTION 1-EKG:

BASIC INTRODUCTION

CHAPTER 1:
Normal Anatomy of Heart:

The human heart is a muscular hollow organ. Its size is approximately equal to the closed fist of a person, but It is responsible for pumping blood throughout the body.

Heart consist of four muscular chambers:

- Right Atrium
- Right Ventricle
- Left Atrium
- Left ventricle

These four chambers are separated by each other through four valves

- Aortic valve
- Pulmonary valve
- Bicuspid valve
- Tricuspid valve

Both ventricles are separated by each other through the interventricular septum

The interatrial septum separates both atria

Four main layers are:

- Pericardium
- Epicardium
- Myocardium
- Endocardium

Four major vessels attaching with heart:

- Pulmonary arteries
- Pulmonary veins
- Aorta
- Superior and Inferior vena cave

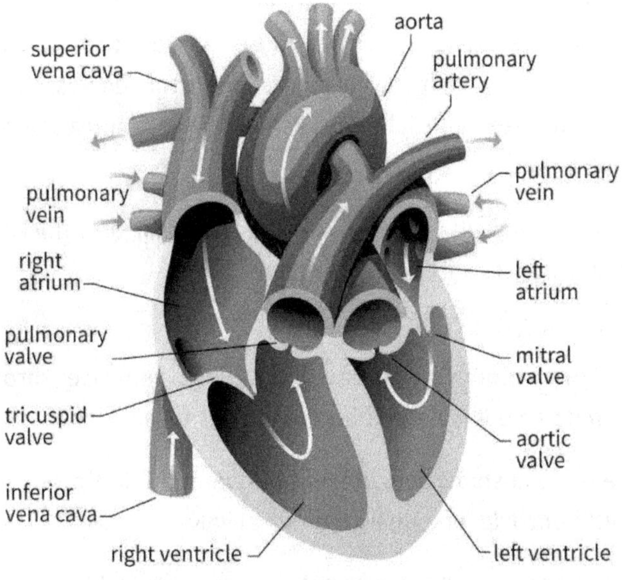

Heart Chambers

Anatomically heart is a single structure, but physiologically heart is divided into two sides; the **right side** and the **left side.**

The right side of the heart is consists of the **right atrium and right ventricle.**

The left side of the heart is consists of the **left atrium and left ventricle.**

The right side and left sides of the heart are anatomically separate by **the atrial septum and the ventricular septum.**

The two sides of the heart are two separate pumps and primarily work independently of each other.

Both atria are smooth-walled low-pressure chambers mainly designed to receive blood from attached vessels.

While both ventricles have thick muscular walls to catch blood from atria and push it with pressure into attached vessels. The walls of the left ventricle are flashy and more muscular than the right ventricle.

The interventricular septum is more muscular and thicker as compared to the interatrial septum.

Heart valves:

The right atrium is separated by Right ventricle through **tricuspid valve.**it is named because it has three cusps

There is a bicuspid valve, present between the left atrium and the left ventricle, known as the mitral valve.

The pulmonary artery originates from the right ventricle, which is guarded by the **Pulmonary valve** While Aorta arises from the left ventricle separated by **Aortic valve.**

The aortic and pulmonic valves are also known as semilunar valves because of their distinct half-moon appearance

The main role of these valves is to prevent the backflow of blood.

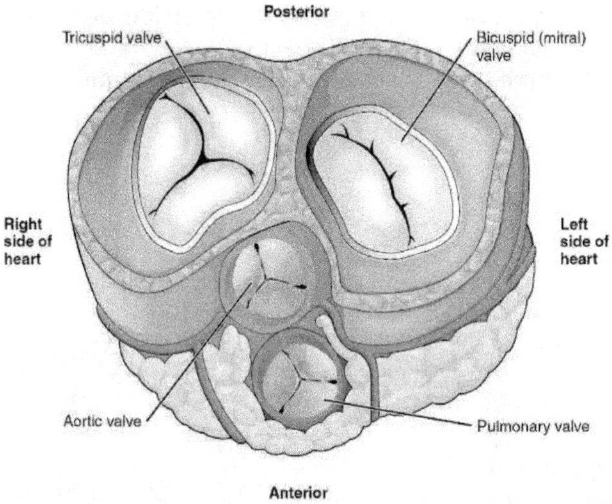

Layers of the Heart

The outermost layer of the heart muscle is known as **Epicardium**. The other name of epicardium is the visceral pericardium.

The **myocardium is the mid-layer of the heart,** which is the thick muscular layer and is responsible for the heart's ability to contract.

The innermost layer is the **endocardium**. This layer of the heart lines the valves and chambers.

The **pericardium** is a loose-fitting fibro serous sac that covers the heart. If we are separating the epicardium, the outermost layer of the heart muscle from the pericardium is a space called the **pericardial space or Pericardial cavity**. Pericardial Space is full of a fluid that acts as a lubricating agent and protects the heart from injuries caused by friction when it is beating.

Phrenic nerve gives neuronal supply the pericardium.

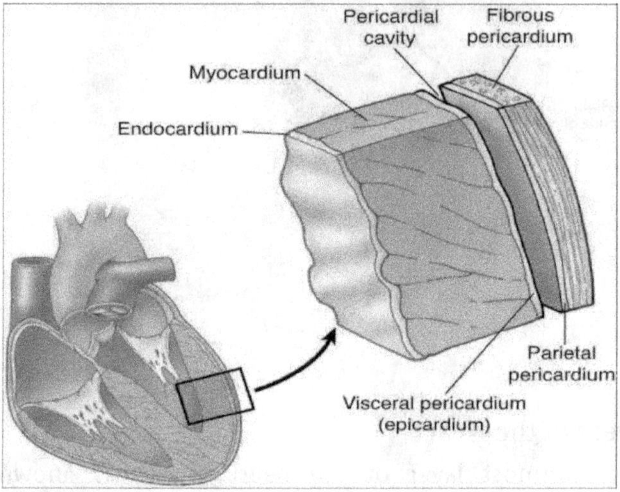

Blood vessels and Circulatory pathway

The right atrium collects the deoxygenated blood from the body through the **superior and inferior venae cavae**.

During diastole, the blood is pushed from the right atrium into the right ventricle through the tricuspid valve.

The blood is then forced out of the right ventricle into the pulmonary circulation via the **pulmonary artery** where it picks up oxygen.

Pulmonary veins carry the oxygenated blood to the left atrium. During ventricular diastole, the blood moves into the left ventricle through the mitral valve.

The left ventricle pumps the oxygen-rich blood throughout the body via **Aorta**

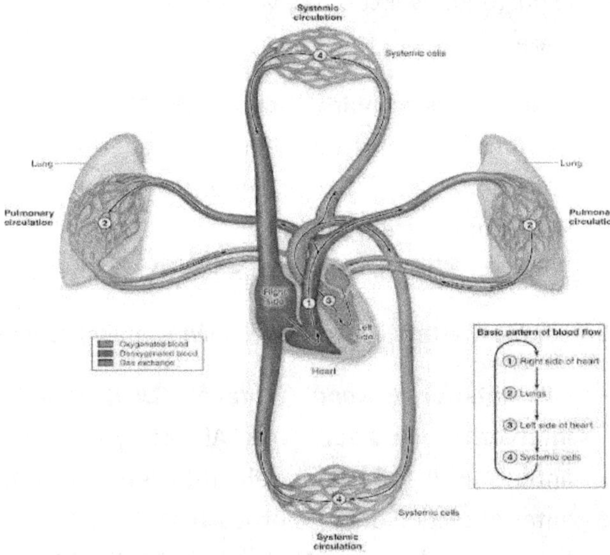

The Coronary Circulation

Although the heart provides oxygenated blood to the whole body, heart muscles itself can't use it directly.so there are some specialized blood vessels for heart muscles known as **coronary vessels.**

The heart muscle receives oxygenated blood by two main vessels:

- **The right coronary artery (RCA)**
- **The left coronary artery (LCA).**

Both arteries arise from the **aortic root (part of Aorta)**. As they travel down the length of the heart, each divide into several branches.

The right coronary artery runs in the coronary sulcus, which is the groove between the atria and the ventricles. It continues down the posterior aspect of the ventricular septum. Its main branches are

- **Posterior descending branch (PDA) or Posterior interventricular artery (PIV)** supplies AV node, posterior part of the interventricular septum, posterior walls of ventricles.
- **The right marginal artery** supplies the right ventricle.

The left coronary artery consists of following main branches

- **Left anterior descending branch (LAD) or Anterior interventricular artery.** The LAD artery perfuses the anterior wall and lateral wall of the left ventricle, the anterior section of the ventricular septum.
- **Left marginal artery (LMA) or Left Obtuse artery.**
- **The circumflex branch (CFX):** It is the branch of the left coronary artery that supplies blood to the left atrium and the posterior and lateral walls of the left ventricle.

Blood enters in coronary arteries in early diastole. These main branches of the coronary arteries typically do not link or anastomose with each other at their ends and are therefore called "end arteries."

This anatomical feature causes significant problems when atherosclerotic lesions develop in the arteries because there is no alternate pathway for the blood to travel.

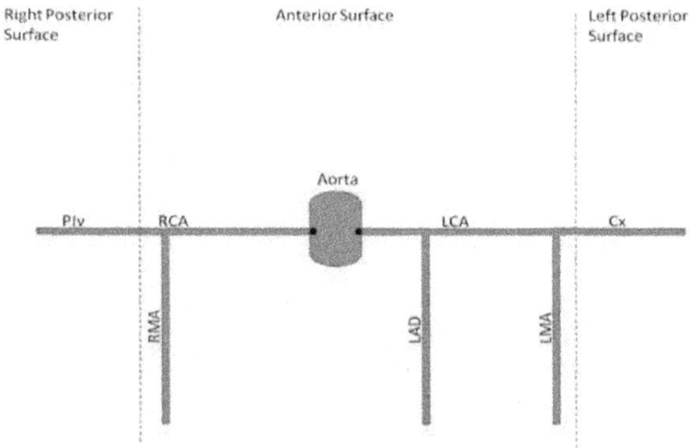

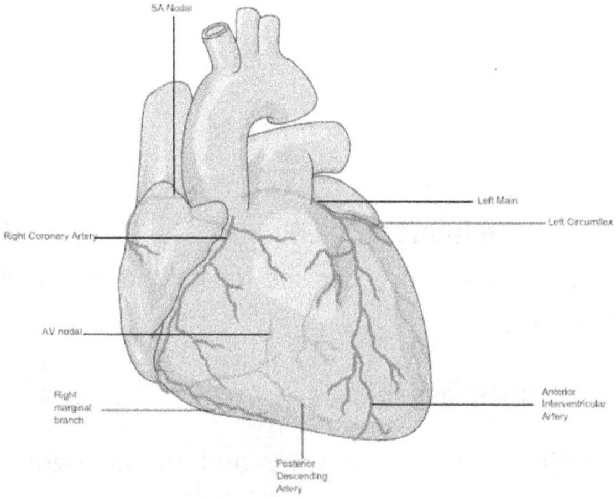

Anatomical Relations

The anatomical position of the human heart is at the level of thoracic vertebrae T5-T8 in the middle mediastinum.

- anteriorly: the body of the sternum and attached costal cartilages; left lung and pleura (apex)
- posteriorly: esophagus, descending thoracic aorta, azygos, and hemiazygos veins, thoracic duct

- superiorly: bifurcation of the main pulmonary trunk
- inferiorly: diaphragm
- laterally: lungs, pleura

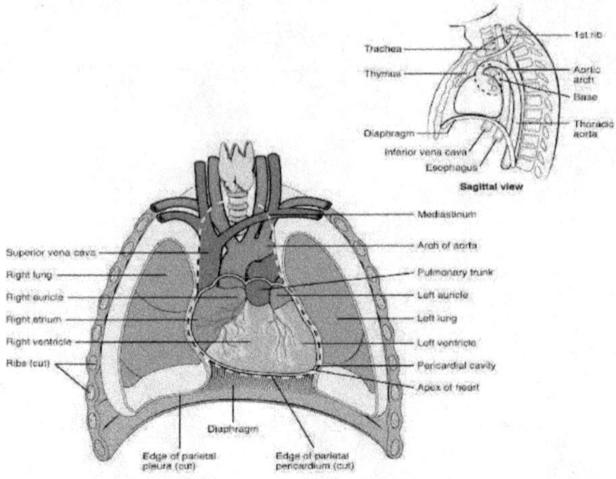

Surfaces of the heart

Anatomically the heart can be described as having the following surfaces:

<u>posterior surface (base):</u>

It is directed upward, backward and to the right, formed mainly by the **left atrium** and little by the right atrium

<u>apex</u>

It is aimed downward, forward and to the left formed mainly by the **left ventricle**

<u>anterior (sternocostal) surface</u>

It is guided forward, upward, and to the left formed mainly by the **right ventricle** inferiorly and right atria superiorly.

inferior (diaphragmatic) surface

It is directed downward, slightly backward formed by **both ventricles'** which rests mainly upon the central tendon of the diaphragm

right surface

It is long and formed by **right atrium** superiorly and **right ventricle** inferiorly

left (pulmonary) surface

It is shorter and rounded; formed mainly by the **left ventricle** and a little superiorly by the left atrium

Borders of the heart

The heart has four borders:

- right border: Inferior vena cava, right atrium, Superior vena cava
- left border: left ventricle, left atrium, pulmonary trunk, and arch of aorta
- inferior border: right ventricle
- superior border: right and left atria, Superior vena cava, ascending aorta and pulmonary trunk

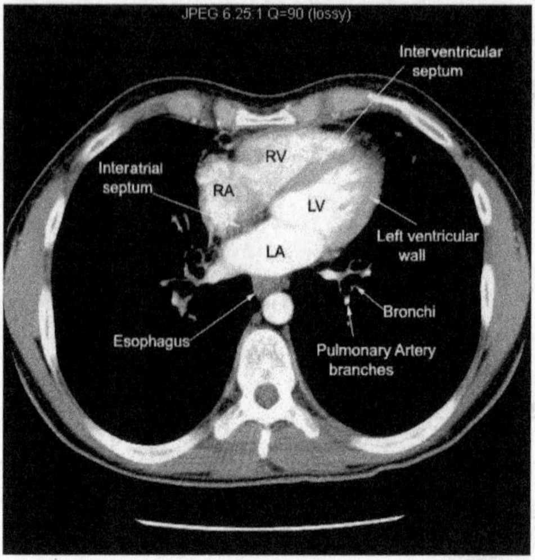

RV is Right ventricle, RA is Right atrium, LA is left atrium, LV is left ventricle

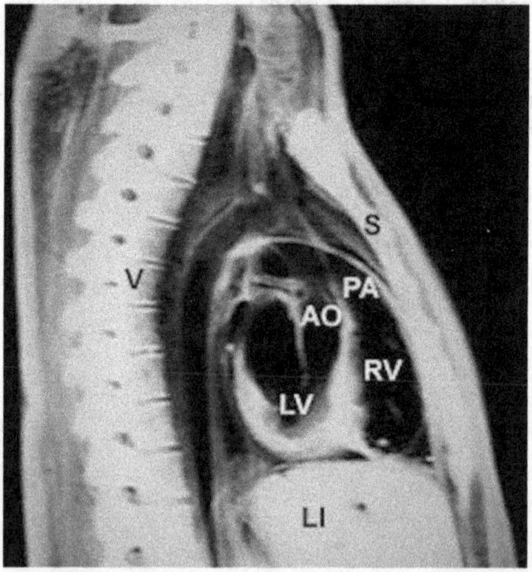

S=sternum, PA=Pulmonary artery, RV=right ventricle, LV=Left ventricle, AO=Aorta, V=Vertebrae, LI=Liver

CHAPTER 2:
Conduction Pathway of heart

The heart's electrical system consists of five structures:

- the sinoatrial (or SA) node,
- the atrioventricular (or AV) node,
- the bundle of His,
- the right and left bundle branches,
- Purkinje fibers.

The conduction system of the heart conducts electrical signals generated usually by the **sinoatrial node**.

The peacemaking signal generated in the sinoatrial node travels through the right atrium to the **atrioventricular node**.

From AV-node, these signals travel down the **Bundle of His.** Through **bundle branches** to the individual **Purkinje fibers** on each side of the heart. When it reaches the endocardium at the apex of the heart, it finally moves to the ventricular epicardium, triggering its contraction. These signals are generated in a regular pattern, which causes contraction of the heart muscle.

This signal initiates contraction, first in the right and left atrium, and then in the right and left ventricles. The right and left atria contracts during atrial systole, as the electrical impulse triggers atrial contraction. While the right and left ventricles contract during ventricular systole. This process lets blood to be pumped throughout the body.

Speed of conduction in different parts of the heart is as in the following order—Purkinje > atria> ventricles > AV node.

Electrical System of the Heart

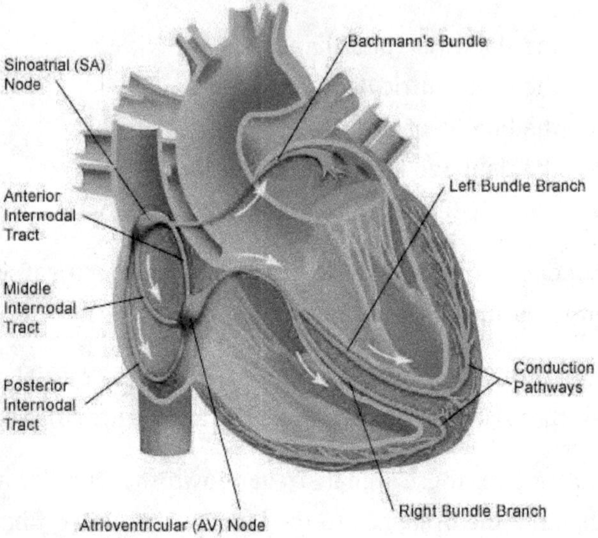

SA-node:

Sino-atrial node or SA node is located in the upper part of the right atrium.

Blood supply is usually from RCA (right coronary artery).

The sinoatrial node (SA node) is the **natural pacemaker** of the heart because it typically initiates each heartbeat and maintains cardiac pace. SA node comprises hundreds of specialized cells that can spontaneously produce an electrical impulse.

The SA node naturally can generate an average of **60 to 100 pulses per minute.** These impulses that travel through the atria by the internodal conduction pathway cause the atria to contract. Both atria get depolarized, as the signal also heads for the AV node.

This electrical activation of the atria, also known as atrial depolarization is represented on the EKG as a **"P" wave.** This is the first wave, or "deflection," on the EKG.

The sinus node is under the control of two parts of the nervous system – the sympathetic and parasympathetic nervous systems

AV-node and bundles:

Atrio-ventricular node or AV node is located in the posteroinferior part of the interatrial septum.

Blood supply is usually from RCA (right coronary artery). It can generate **40-60 impulses per minute** without SA node

There is a delay of 100-msec in the conduction of electric signals at the AV node. This delay allows atria to contract first, then ventricles and provides sufficient time for ventricular filling. The delay in the AV node forms a significant part of **the PR segment on the ECG.** The PR segment also represents a portion of atrial repolarization.

From AV-node, the **bundle of His** conducts the electrical impulse through to the **bundle branches.** The electrical stimulus travels through the bundle branches to the **Purkinje fibers.** This electric impulse depolarizes the myocardial cells of both ventricles, which is described as ventricular depolarization. Ventricular depolarization is signified on the EKG as the **QRS complex, which is the second deflection on EKG.** Ventricles can beat independently without SA and AV node at the rate of **20-40 impulses** per minute.

The T wave is the third deflection on the EKG. The T wave represents ventricular repolarization. The ventricles must repolarize or recharge themselves or normalize again before the next cardiac cycle can begin. **ST-segment** also marks ventricular repolarization.

Atria also repolarizes, but the QRS complex masks atrial repolarization wave.

In a few cases, a new wave can be seen at the end of the T wave, which is known as a U wave. Its origin is uncertain.

Summary:

- P wave—atrial depolarization. QRS complex conceals the atrial repolarization waves.
- PR interval—It is the time from the start of atrial depolarization to start of ventricular depolarization
- QRS complex—ventricular depolarization.
- QT interval—ventricular depolarization, automated contraction of the ventricles, ventricular repolarization.
- T wave—represents ventricular repolarization.
- J point—the junction in the middle of the end of the QRS complex and the start of ST-segment.
- ST-segment—isoelectric, ventricles depolarized.
- U wave—of uncertain origin.

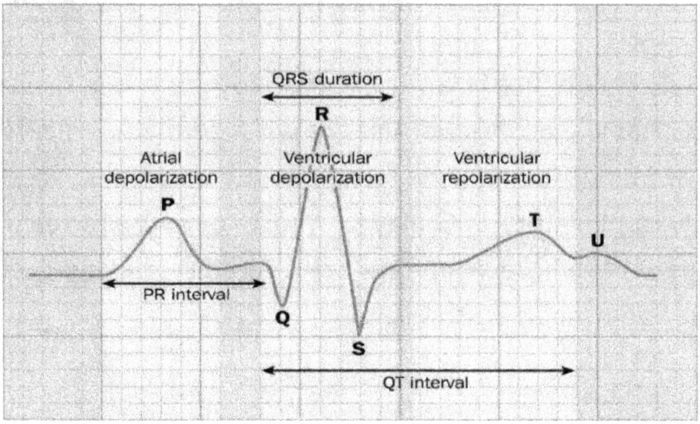

CHAPTER 3:
Basis of EKG:

Types of ECG

There are three main types of ECG:

The type of ECG will depend on symptoms and the heart problem suspected.

- **A resting ECG** – It is carried out while you're lying down in a comfortable position
- **a stress or exercise ECG** – It is carried out while you're using an exercise bike or treadmill. An exercise ECG may be recommended if symptoms are triggered by physical activity.
- **An ambulatory ECG –** the electrodes are linked to a small portable machine worn at the waist so that the heart can be monitored at home for one or more days.

  An ambulatory ECG may be more appropriate for those patients whose symptoms are unpredictable and occur in random, short episodes.

EKG Machine:

Electrocardiographs are recorded by mechanical devices that consist of a set of electrodes connected to a central unit. Nowadays, ECG machines are portable and commonly include a screen, keyboard, and printer on a small wheeled cart.

Recording an ECG is a harmless and painless procedure. A conduction jelly is applied to the skin before attaching the ECG leads. This jelly increase in the conductivity of leads. Before starting the recording, any metal ornaments should be removed because they may cause interference in recording signals.

New modern ECG machines consist of automated interpretation algorithms. These algorithms allow these machines to calculate elements such as the PR axis, PR interval, QT interval, corrected QT (QTc) interval, QRS axis, rhythm, and more. But there are chances of errors in interpretation by machines, so every physician should know how to interpret EKG.

ECG Paper:

The ECG paper is a ribbon-like piece of graph paper with large and small gratings.

On the horizontal axis (x-axis), each 1 mm square (the smallest square) represents 0.04 seconds, and each large square (5 mm) represents 0.2 seconds.

On the vertical axis (y-axis), each large square represents 0.5 mV.

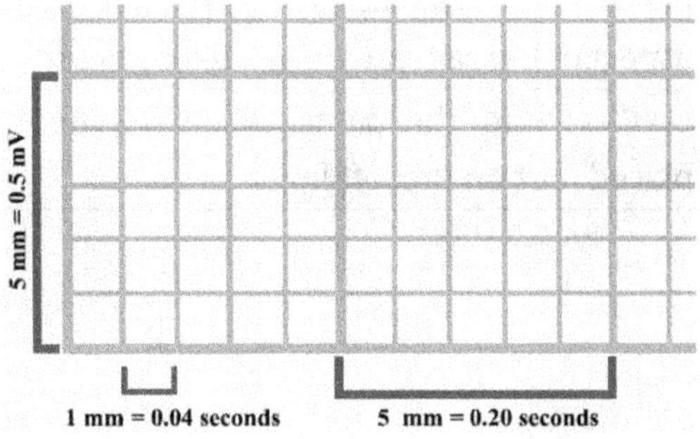

EKG LEADS:

As we have already discussed, the heart has a unique ability to produce spontaneous electrical potential, which causes the contraction of cardiac muscles and makes the heart pump blood. To capture the cardiac activity, specific Electrodes are used known as **LEADS.** These Electrodes are the actual conductive pads attached to the body surface. Any pair of leads can calculate the electrical potential difference between the two successive locations of attachment. Each point is meant to record electrical activity from a different position on the heart muscle. This arrangement of leads permits an experienced interpreter to see the heart from many different angles.

Usually, ten electrodes are attached to the body to form 12 ECG leads. Leads are divided into three types: limb, augmented limb, and precordial or chest.

Limb leads:

• RA=On the right arm, avoiding thick muscles.
• LA=Placed In the same site where RA was placed, but on the left arm.
• RL=On the right leg, the lower end of the inner aspect of the calf muscle. (Avoid bony prominences)
• LL=Placed In the same position where RL was placed, but on the left leg.

Chest leads:

• V1= to the right of the sternum, In the fourth intercostal space,	• V2= to the left of the sternum, Positioned In the fourth intercostal space
• V3=Placed amongst leads V2 and V4.	• V4= in the mid-clavicular line, In the left fifth intercostal space
• V5=Placed horizontally even with V4, in the left anterior axillary line.	• V6=Placed horizontally even with V4 and V5 in the mid-axillary line

- .

Leads aVR, aVL, and aVF are designated as the **augmented limb leads**. They are derived from the three electrodes of leads I, II, and III.

There are specific **specialized leads** as well; for example, Posterior leads (V7 to V9) may be used to establish the presence of a posterior myocardial infarction. A Lewis lead that requires an electrode at the right sternal border in the second intercostal space is used to study pathological rhythms arising in the right atrium. An esophageal lead can be inserted into a part of the esophagus to record signals from the left atrium, especially in cases of arrhythmias.

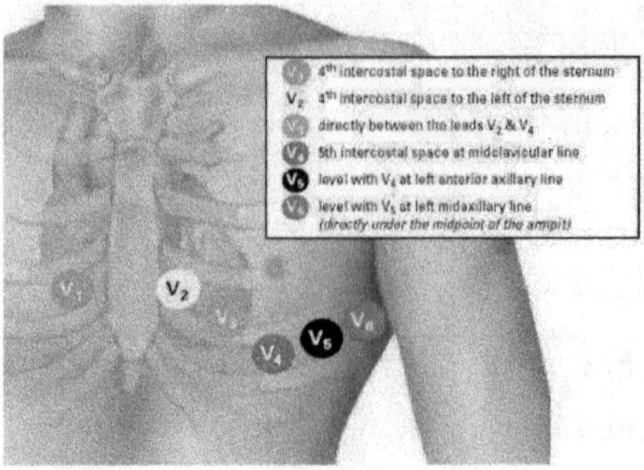

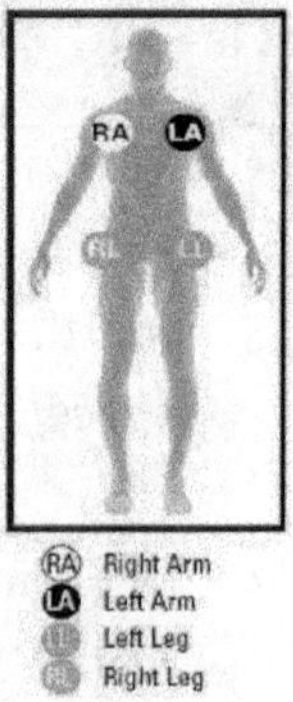

These 12 ECG leads have a unique way of representing the picture of the heart.

Category	Leads	Activity
Inferior leads	II, III, and aVF	Look at electrical activity from the inferior surface (diaphragmatic) surface of the heart.
Lateral leads	I, aVL, V_5 and V_6	Look at the electrical activity from the lateral wall of the left ventricle
Septal leads	V_1 and V_2	Look at electrical activity from the septal surface of the heart (interventricular septum)
Anterior leads	V_3 and V_4	Look at electrical activity from the anterior wall of the right and left ventricles (Sternocostal surface of the heart)

PORTION 2:

HOW TO INTERPRET EKG

CHAPTER 4: CHECKLIST FOR ECG INTERPRETATION

Following is the checklist for EKG interpretation

- **Clinical data**
- **Standardization**
- **Heart rate**
- **Rhythm**
- **Axis**
- **P-wave, QRS complex, T-waves**
- **St segment**
- **PR-interval, QT-interval. RR- interval**

We must go through each step one by one, looking for any possible abnormality.

In case of any abnormality, it's crucial to identify in which lead and sister leads it is present.

Clinical Data

Clinical data recording is vital for EKG. There should be proper data regarding

NAME

AGE

SEX

MEDICAL DIAGNOSIS/MOST PROBABLE DIAGNOSIS

MEDICATIONS IN USE

PROCEDURES DONE SO FAR

ANY ASSOCIATED MEDICAL CONDITION

Time (EKG was done)

EKG technologist:

Standardized recording

ECG tracings are recorded on grid paper. At the horizontal axis of the **EKG, paper time is** recorded. The black marks at the top indicate 3-second intervals.

Each second is marked by five large grid blocks (total 15 large blocks in 3 seconds). Thus each large block equals 0.2 seconds. Within the large blocks, there are five small blocks, each representing 0.04 seconds.

The vertical axis records EKG amplitude (voltage). Two large blocks equal 1millivolt, and One large block is equal to 0.5 millivolts (mV). Each small-block equals 0.1 mV.

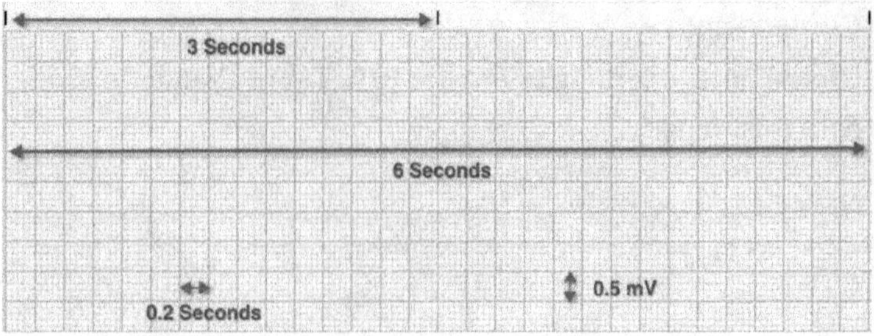

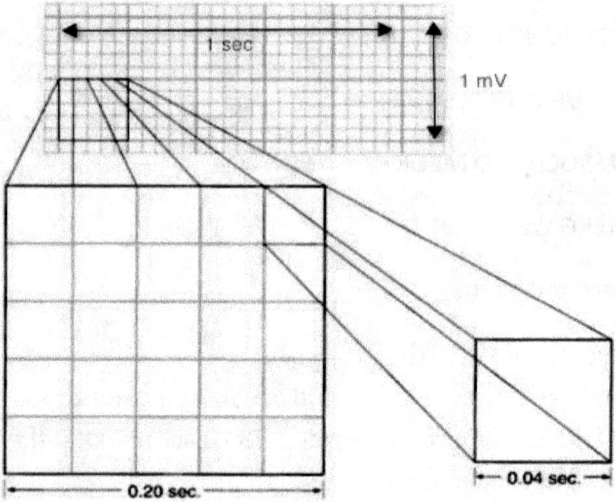

Each small box is 1 mm. Each large box is of 5mm

Electrocardiogram Calibration

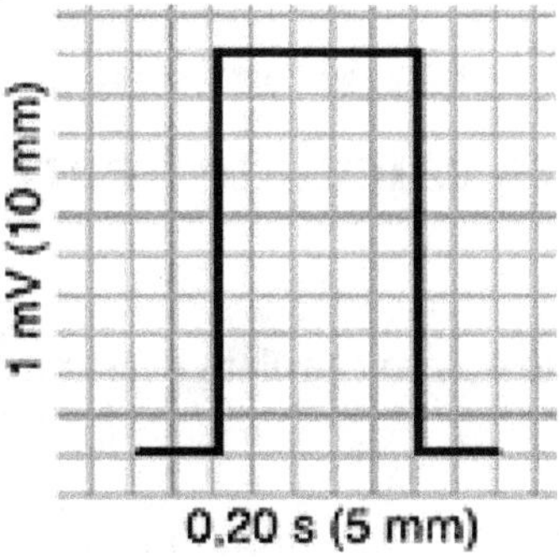

The electrocardiograph automatically performs calibration at the beginning of the electrocardiogram recording.

An electrical signal of 1 mv is sent for 0.2 s, results in the recording of a rectangular shape with a 10 mm height and 5 mm width on the graph paper.

This image lets us know the calibration used during the recorded EKG.

The speed of the paper or amplitude can be adjusted in conditions where the QRS voltages are either too high or too low.

CHAPTER 5:
How to calculate heart rate:

The most accurate way to calculate heart rate is by measuring the R-R interval.

The R-R interval is the space from one R wave to the next R wave. When evaluating the R-R interval, take the start of one QRS complex, and count the number of "little boxes" up to the beginning of the next QRS complex. Divide this number into 1500. This technique of calculating the heart rate is acceptable only if the heart rate is regular. Or the heart rate is 300 divided by the number of large squares between the QRS complexes.

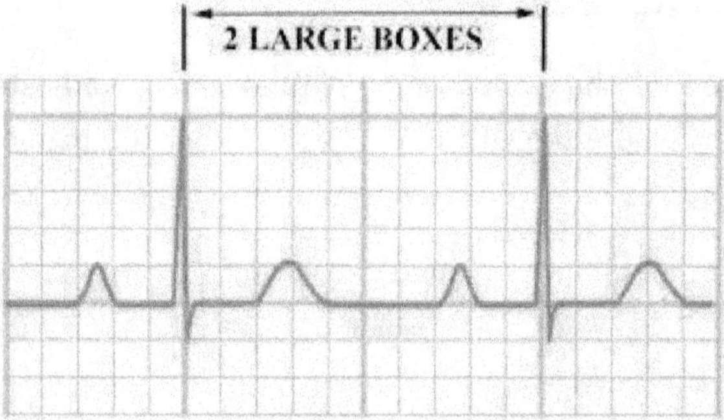

Heart Rate = 300 divided by 2 large boxes = 150 bpm

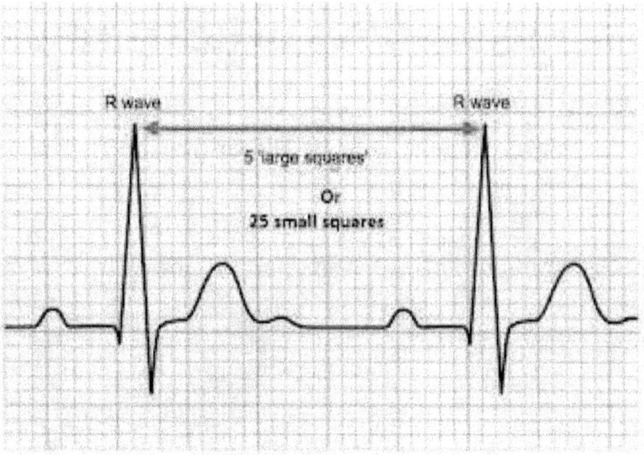

Heart rate $= \frac{1500}{25} =$ **60 per minute**

Lead II OR **rhythm lead** is considered as a perfect lead to calculate heart rate.

In **leads II, III, aVF"** P" wave is upright, so it's effortless to get recognized.

The sinus node naturally adjusts and controls the heart at a rate of 60 to 100 beats

per minute (bpm), which is called **sinus rhythm**, or normal sinus rhythm.

AGE SPAN	**HEART RATE (bpm)**
Less than 1 month	120-160
1-12 months	80-140
12 months - 2 years	80-130
2-6 years	75-120
6-12 years	75-110
More than 12 years	60-100

Abnormalities of heart rate:

Sinus Bradycardia:

When the sinus rate is **below 60 bpm**, this is called **sinus Bradycardia.**

A normal impulse is generated from SA node but at a slower rate.

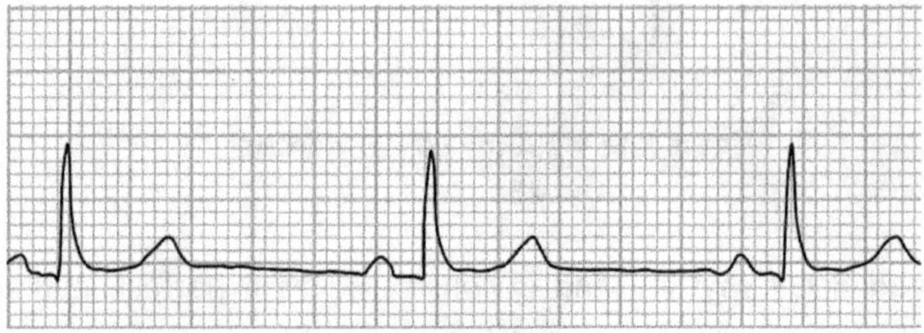

Sinus bradycardia signifies a relative imbalance in the healthy sympathetic/ parasympathetic balance of the heart. There are two leading causes of sinus bradycardia: (1) decreased sympathetic activity or (2) increased parasympathetic activity.

Sympathetic activity decreases while taking drugs (that block the sympathetic nervous system in the treatment of hypertension) coronary artery disease, and heart failure.

The vagal response is a common cause of increased parasympathetic activity. The vagal response can occur due to gastrointestinal (GI) stimulation during nausea, vomiting, and drug treatment.

Some causes of sinus bradycardia:

- Beta-blocker therapy
- Vagal response (increased parasympathetic tone)
- Hypothyroidism
- Athlete's conditioning

Sinus tachycardia:

When the sinus rate is higher than 100bpm, it is called **sinus tachycardia**. A normal impulse is generated from SA node but at a faster pace.

It is either due to an increase in the sympathetic stimulation or a decrease in the parasympathetic stimulation.

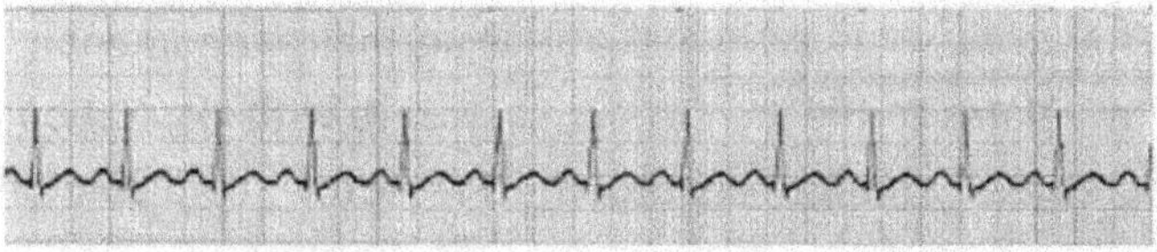

Some causes of sinus tachycardia:

- Shock
- Heart failure
- Bleeding
- Infection
- Hyperthyroidism
- Pulmonary embolism
- Sympathomimetic drug therapy

- Anxiety
- Hypoglycemia
- Hypoxia

When the heart rate fluctuates by more than 10%, the rhythm is called **sinus arrhythmia.** When the interval between QRS complexes are irregular, the best way to assess the heart rate is by tallying the number of QRS complexes in a 6-second block of time and multiplying that number by 10.

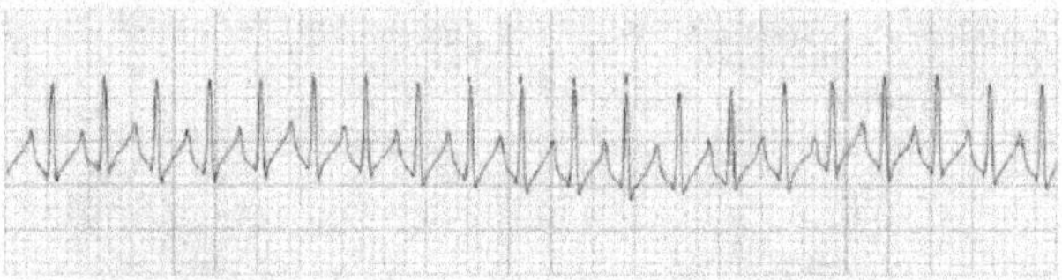

Respiratory sinus arrhythmias: (RSA)

Respiratory sinus arrhythmia is a normal phenomenon; the term relates to the increase in heart rate with inspiration and decreases during expiration. Premotor cardioinhibitory parasympathetic neurons (CPNs) in the brainstem controls the heart rate, and RSA is mediated in part by central respiratory modulation of CPN activity through VAGUS nerve. During the respiratory cycle, inspiration inhibits vagal tone leading to an increase in sinus rate, while expiration increases vagal tone resulting in a decreased rate.

The R-R interval on an ECG is reduced during inspiration and prolonged during expiration.

Respiratory sinus arrhythmia is observed more frequently in children than adults and tends to fade away as they get older. If a respiratory sinus arrhythmia is found in older individuals, it's often associated with heart disease or another heart condition

As the heart speeds up, for example, during exercise, the heart rate rhythm tends to become more regular.

Respiratory sinus arrhythmias (RSA) is a sign of a healthy heart and normal cardiovascular system. It is not a pathological finding.

Relation between ECG and Respiration Series

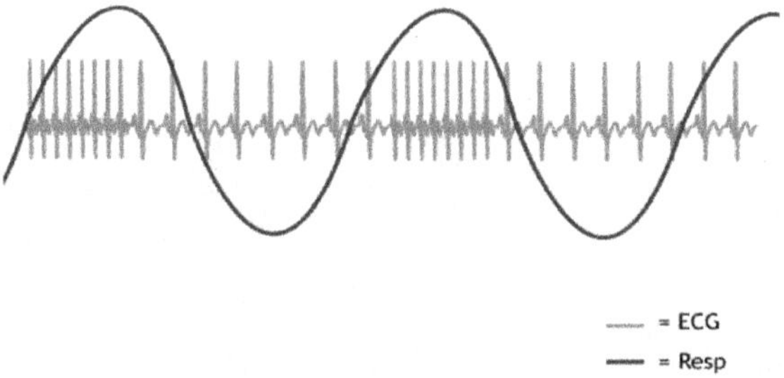

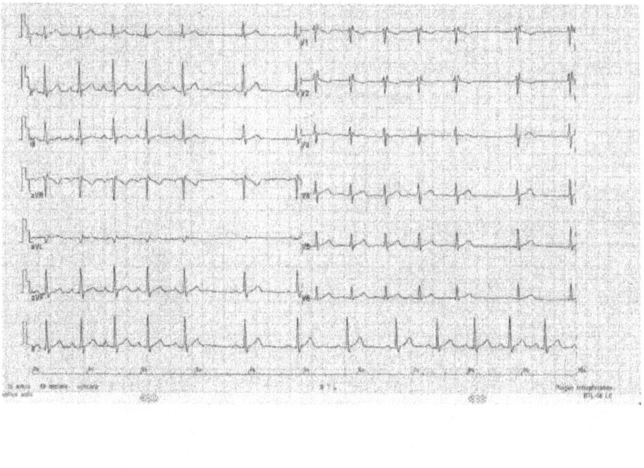

In the above EKG focus on lead II, the rhythm lead, you will see the variation in heart rate and R-R interval that is phasic, but if look at P-wave and its relation with QRS complex, it will be normal.

CHAPTER 6:
Heart Rhythm assessment

SA node is the pacemaker of the heart. It determines the rate and pace at which the heart will beat.

On EKG, if you see a normal P wave before a QRS complex, the QRS complex is of standard shape and duration, and T-waves follow it, It means this Normal electrical activity is generated by SA node.

If P-waves or QRS complexes are at regular intervals from each other, this means that the SA node is generating impulses at a consistent pace; this is called **sinus rhythm.** But if either the pulse produces at irregular pace OR originate from somewhere else other than SA node, it is known as **Arrhythmias.**

On EKG strip P-wave and QRS complexes will be at irregular intervals, OR R-R distance will be different among different QRS complexes.

The keys to diagnosing abnormalities of heart rhythm are:

- The P waves –Find the lead in which they are most prominent (II, III, aVF).
- The relationship between the P waves and the QRS complexes – there should be one P wave per QRS complex.
- The width of the QRS complexes

- Look for the shape of QRS complexes. Is there any with the unusual shape?
- What is the shape of a T-wave?

Arrhythmias, based on origin, can be

- Supraventricular
- Ventricular

Supraventricular tachycardia

Supraventricular tachycardia (SVT) is also known as paroxysmal supraventricular tachycardia. It is an episodic condition with a sudden onset and cessation.

Their specific site of origin more accurately categorizes the following types of supraventricular tachycardias.

Sinoatrial origin: Sinoatrial nodal reentrant tachycardia (SNRT)

Atrial origin:

- Ectopic (unifocal) atrial tachycardia (EAT)
- Multifocal atrial tachycardia (MAT)
- Atrial fibrillation with rapid ventricular response
- Atrial flutter with fast ventricular response

Fibrillation and flutter are usually not categorized as SVT unless there is a rapid ventricular response.

Atrioventricular origin OR junctional tachycardia:

- AV nodal reentrant tachycardia (AVNRT) also known as junctional reciprocating tachycardia (JRT)
- Permanent (or persistent) junctional reciprocating tachycardia (PJRT)
- AV reciprocating tachycardia (AVRT) – visible or hidden accessory pathway (including Wolff-Parkinson-White syndrome)
- Junctional ectopic tachycardia (JET)

Sinoatrial node reentrant tachycardia (SANRT)

Sinoatrial node reentrant tachycardia (SANRT) is produced by a reentry circuit located close to the SA node, causing a P-wave of standard shape and size (morphology). P-wave falls before a regular, narrow QRS complex. It cannot be distinguished on EKG from sinus tachycardia unless the sudden onset is observed (or recorded on a continuous monitoring device). Heart rate is between 100-150 beats. Its quick response to vagal maneuvers may sometimes distinguish it from other tachycardias.

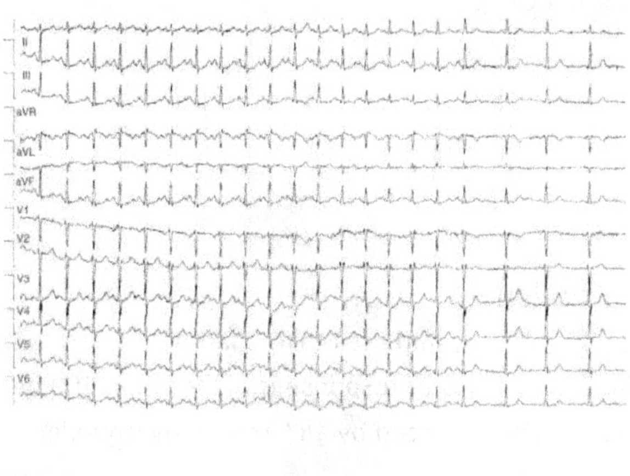

Atrial tachycardia:

Atrial tachycardia (AT) is supraventricular tachycardia (SVT). It is of a regular rhythm at a rate of 160 to 260. Usually, the P wave is absent, if present, appears differently from the normal P-wave. The heart rate increases from 91 to more than 160 bpm. Atrial tachycardia is usually related to increased sympathetic activity. It can be seen in both normal and abnormal hearts.

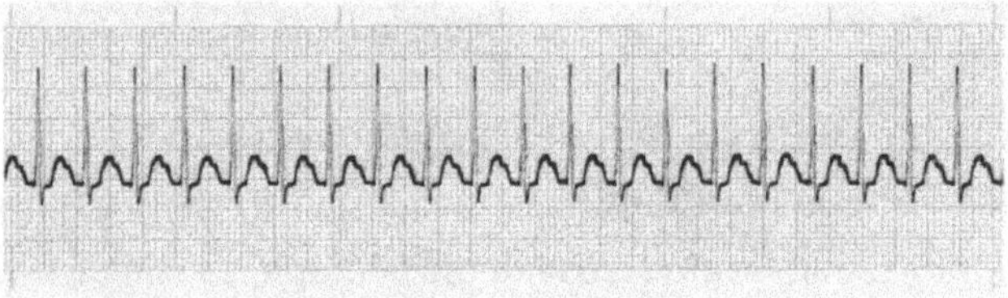

Multifocal atrial tachycardia (MAT)

In MAT, impulses originate irregularly and rapidly from different points in atria. Tachycardia starting from at least three ectopic foci within the atria is recognized by P-waves of at least three different shapes that all fall before irregular, narrow QRS complexes. This rhythm is mostly seen in older adults with COPD.

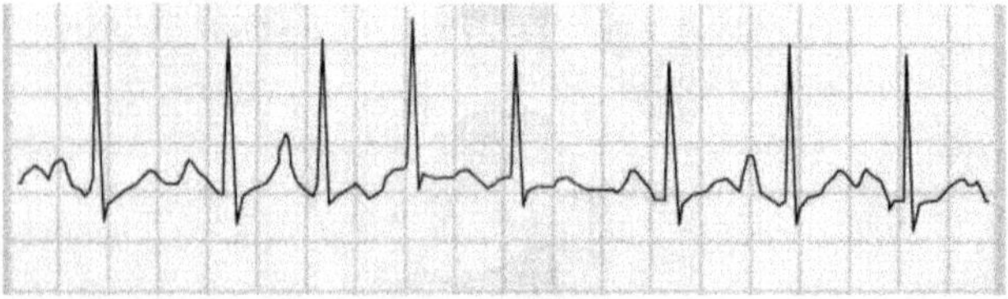

Atrial fibrillation:

In Atrial fibrillation, impulses take chaotic, random pathways in atria. The ventricular response is higher than 100 beats per minute. It is characterized by an "irregularly irregular rhythm" both in its atrial and ventricular depolarizations and is recognized by its fibrillatory atrial waves. In EKG, P-waves are absent, and QRS complexes are irregular and narrow.

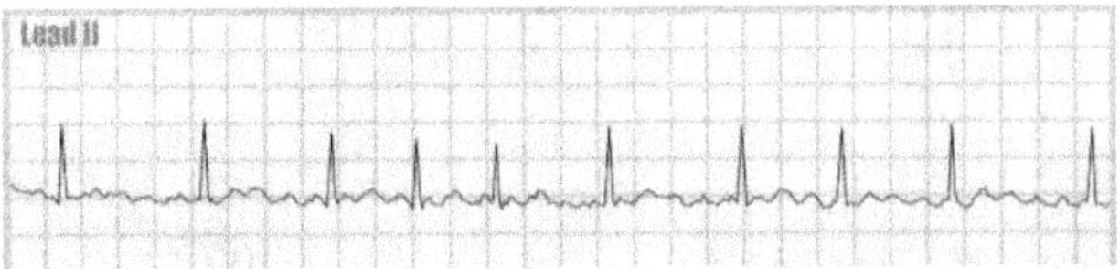

Atrial flutter:

It is caused by a re-entry rhythm in the atria, with a steady atrial rate of about 300 beats per minute. On the ECG, this seems like a line of "sawtooth" waves before the QRS complex. The AV cannot conduct 300 beats per minute, so the P-wave to QRS complex ratio is usually 2:1 or 4:1 pattern. Because the rate of P to QRS is typically consistent, A-flutter is often regular in comparison to atrial fibrillation. Atrial flutter is also not primarily a tachycardia unless the ventricular response is higher than 100 beats per minute.

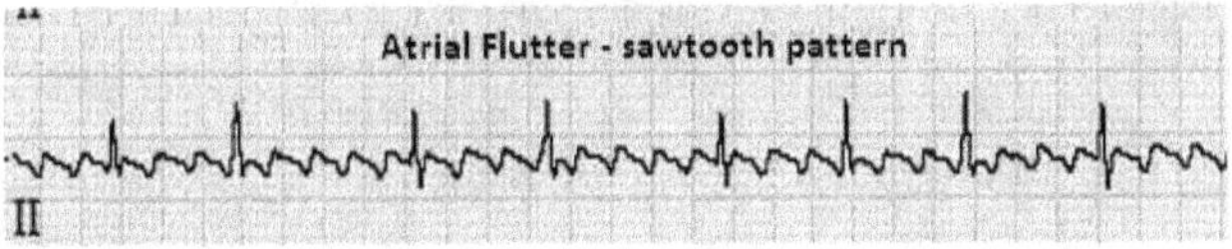

AV nodal reentrant tachycardia (AVNRT):

It involves a reentry circuit forming within the AV node. There is retrograde conduction of impulses leading to backward (retrograde) conducted P-wave buried within or occurring just after the regular, narrow QRS complexes.

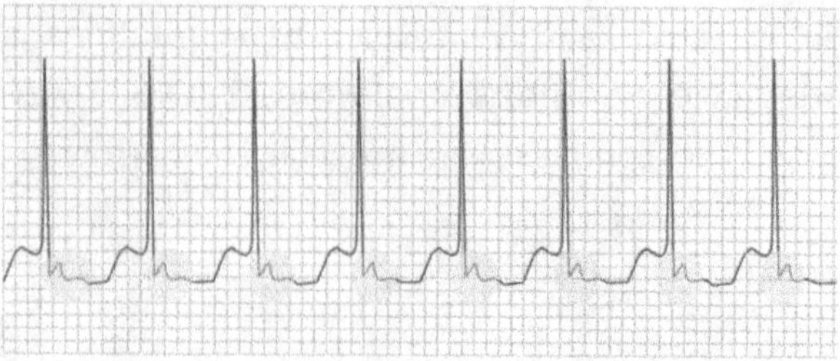

Atrioventricular reciprocating tachycardia (AVRT):

It also results from a reentry circuit, but due to one physically much bigger than AVNRT. One part of the circuit is usually the AV node, and the other is an abnormal accessory pathway (muscular connection) starting from the atria to the ventricle. It has two types, Orthodromic AVRT and Antidromic AVRT.

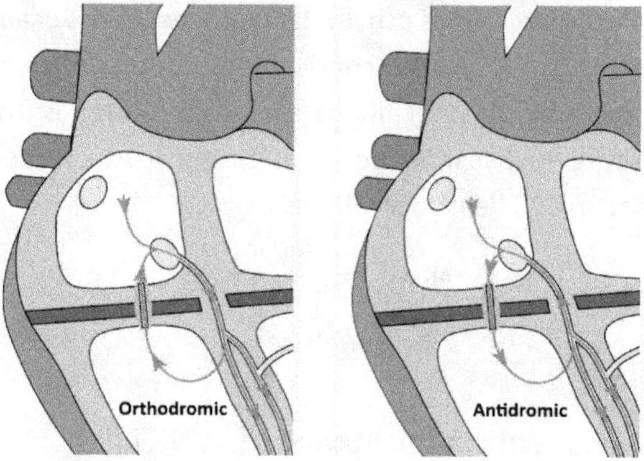

Orthodromic AVRT:

In orthodromic AVRT, atrial impulses are led down through the AV node and retrogradely re-enter the atrium via the accessory pathway. A distinguishing feature of orthodromic AVRT is an inverted P-wave (relative to a sinus P wave), which follows each of its regular, narrow QRS complexes, due to retrograde conduction. Its most common type of SVT.

Antidromic AVRT:

In this condition, atrial impulses are conducted down through the accessory pathway and re-enter the atrium retrogradely via the AV node. As the accessory pathway begins impulse transmission in the ventricles, but beyond the bundle of His, that is why the QRS complex in antidromic AVRT is wider than usual. It is a very uncommon condition.

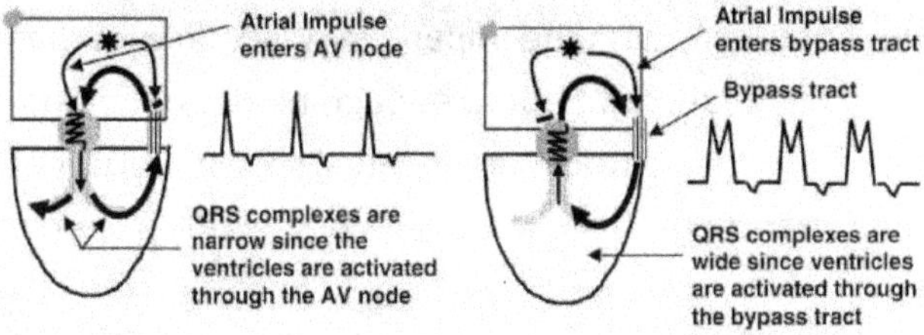

A. Orthodromic AVRT B. Antidromic AVRT

Junctional ectopic tachycardia (JET)

It is a rare tachycardia caused by increased automaticity of the AV node itself initiating frequent heartbeats. On the ECG, junctional tachycardia often describes as abnormally shaped P-waves, which may fall anywhere concerning to a regular, narrow QRS complex. There is retrograde as well as antegrade transmission of impulse resulting in inverted and absent P-waves in EKG. AV node produces pulses at the rate of 40-60/min. It is frequently due to drug toxicity.

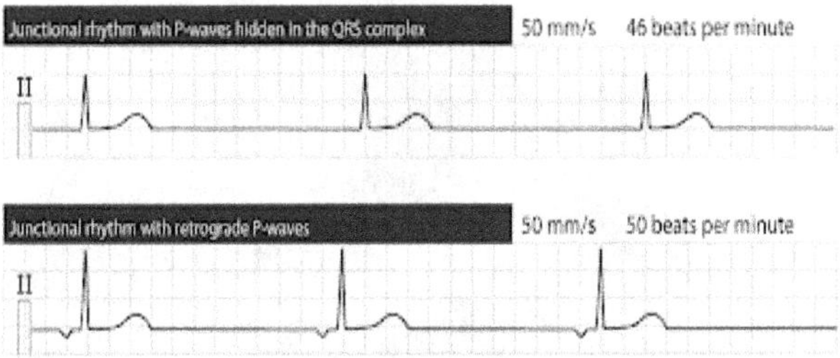

Ventricular tachycardia

Ventricular tachycardia or ventricular fibrillation is a heart rhythm disorder (arrhythmia) caused by irregular electrical signals arising from ventricles (the lower chambers of the heart). In ventricular tachycardia (V-tach or VT), abnormal electrical signals originating from the ventricles cause the heart to beat faster than usual, 100 or even more beats a minute, out of sync with the upper chambers(atria). When that happens, the heart can't pump enough blood to the body and lungs because the ventricles are beating so fast and out of sync with each other that they don't have time to fill properly.

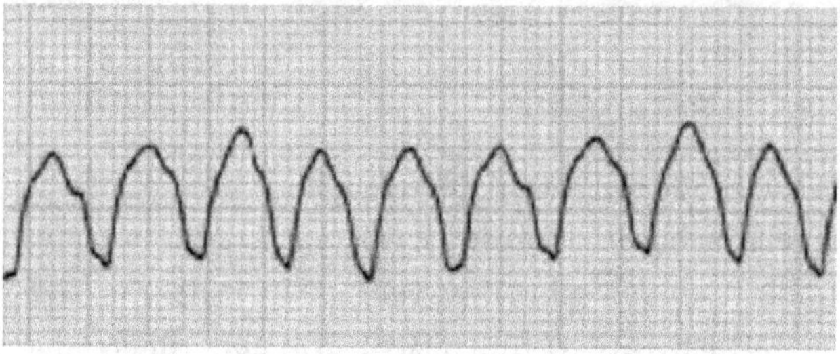

CHAPTER 7:
ELECTRICAL AXIS:

As we have already discussed that the electrical activity of the heart begins from the sinoatrial (SA) node then extends to the atrioventricular (AV) node. It then spreads along with the bundle of his and then Purkinje fibers to trigger contractions of ventricles.

So when watching the heart from the front, the direction of depolarization is from 10 o'clock to 5 o'clock. (starting from the base to the apex of the heart). Directed downwards towards the left.

The general direction of depolarization is known as the cardiac axis, which is captured by limb leads I, II, and III and Leads aVR, aVL, and aVF, which are the augmented limb leads.

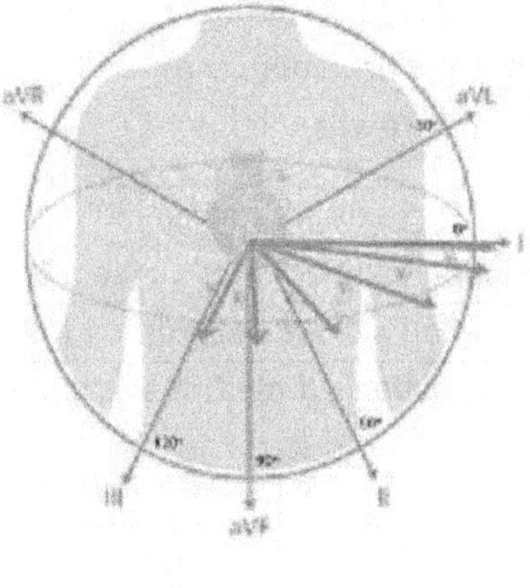

In the above figure lead, II is at 5 o clock position, and lead aVR is at 10 o clock position.

So limb leads are capturing the whole process of depolarization from base to apex of the heart (downwards towards left). The spread of depolarization would be heading in the direction of leads I, II, and III. As a result, there would be a positive deflection in all these leads with lead II being the most positive (it's at 5 o'clock position).

And the most negative deflection in lead aVR, because lead aVR is observing the heart in the opposite direction to lead II.

As we all know, the depolarization of ventricles is marked by the QRS complex so that it will be our major landmark on EKG for the determination of axis.

There are five main electrical axis classifications:

- normal axis
- left axis deviation (LAD)
- right axis deviation (RAD)
- extreme axis deviation, and
- indeterminate axis

Normal Axis =If QRS axis is between -30° and +90°.
Left Axis Deviation =If QRS axis is < than -30°.
Right Axis Deviation = If the QRS axis is > than +90°.
Extreme Axis Deviation = If the QRS axis is between -90° and 180°

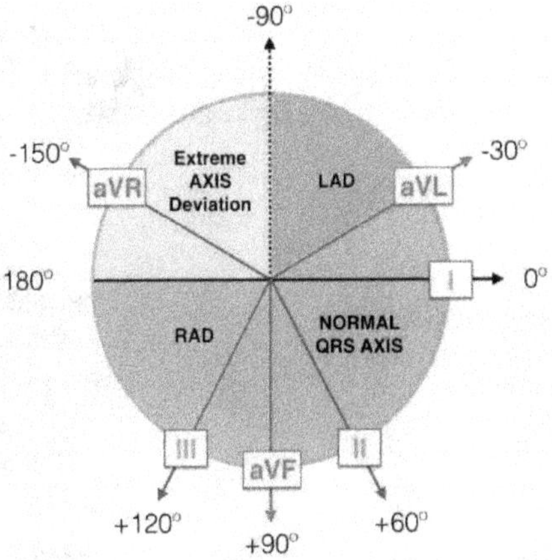

<u>There are multiple methods to calculate the electrical axis.</u>

- The Quadrant Method – (I,aVF)
- Three lead analysis – (I, II,aVF)
- Isoelectric Lead analysis

The Quadrant Method:

The most efficient way to estimate the axis is to look at LEAD I and LEAD aVF.

Observe the QRS complex in each lead and determine if it is Positive, Isoelectric (Equiphasic) or Negative

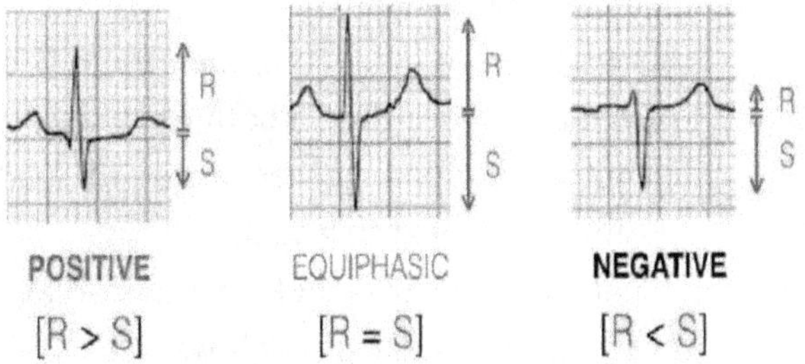

Lead 1	Lead aVF	Quadrant	Axis
POSITIVE	POSITIVE	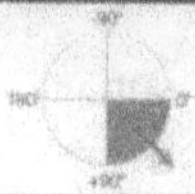	**Normal Axis** (0 to +90°)
POSITIVE	**NEGATIVE**	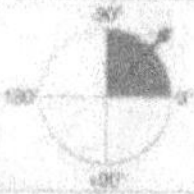	****Possible LAD** (0 to -90°)
NEGATIVE	POSITIVE	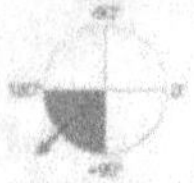	**RAD** (+90° to 180°)
NEGATIVE	**NEGATIVE**	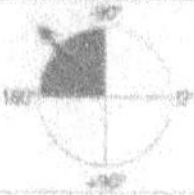	**Extreme Axis** (-90° to 180°)

Three lead methods:

The main **QRS complexes** to calculate axis are those in **leads I, II, and aVF**. The positive ends of these three leads fall in the normal axis region. The positive ends of leads I, II, and aVF are 0 degrees, +60 degrees, and +90 degrees, respectively. To simplify, if all three of these leads have positive QRS complexes, the axis is normal.

I) If the net QRS deflection is positive in both leads I and II, the QRS axis is normal.

II) If the net QRS deflection is positive in the lead I, but negative in the lead II, then there is Left Axis Deviation. Notice that in both examples, lead aVF is not required. In other words, if lead, I am positive, look next to lead II.

III) if lead I am negative, look next to lead aVF. If it is positive, then the axis is rightward

IV) if lead I and aVF are both is negative, then there is the extreme axis.

This methodology is summarized in the following table

	Lead I	Lead II	Lead aVF
NORMAL AXIS (0° TO+90°)	+	+	+
LAD (PHYSIOLOGICAL 0° TO -30°)	+		-
LAD (PATHOLOGICAL -30° TO -90°)	+	-	-
RAD (+90° TO 180°)	-	+	+
EXTREME AXIS (-90° TO 180°)	-	-	-

The Isoelectric Lead

This method allows for a more precise estimation of the QRS axis. Locate the most isoelectric limb lead along the frontal plane.

Key Principles

-If the QRS is POSITIVE in any provided lead, the axis points is roughly the same direction as this lead.

-If the QRS is NEGATIVE in the provided lead, the axis point is roughly the opposite direction as this lead.

-If the QRS is ISOELECTRIC or equiphasic) in any provided lead (positive deflection = negative deflection), the axis is at 90° to this lead.

Step 1: Find the isoelectric lead.

The isoelectric (equiphasic) lead is the lead with a net amplitude of zero. It could be either:

-A biphasic QRS where the height of R wave= depth of Q or S wave.

-A flat-line QRS with no noticeable features.

Step 2: Find the positive leads.

Look for the leads with the highest R waves (or most significant R/S ratios)

Step 3: Calculate the QRS axis.

If the QRS axis is at 90° to the isoelectric lead, it is pointing towards the direction of the positive leads.

Explanation with an example:

- Look at EKG below
- CHECK ONLY LEADS I, II, III and aVR, aVL, and aVF
- aVL is the lead that has the most isoelectric QRS complex. (read again the definition of the isoelectric complex from above)
- lead II has tallest R waves among these six leads
- Axis at aVL lead is -30° while at lead II its +60 °
- The normal QRS axis lies in between two values of -30° and +90°.
- So this EKG has a normal axis.

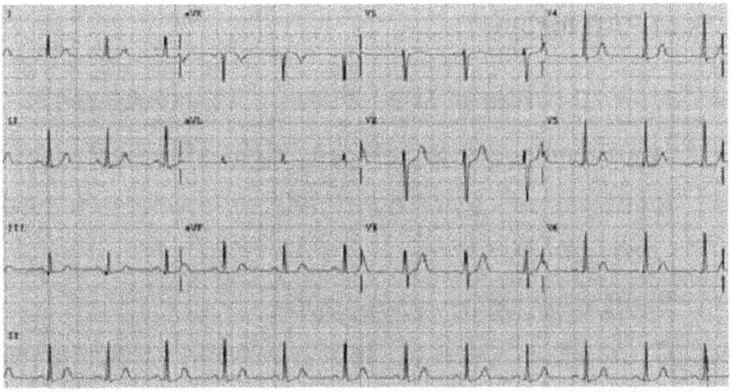

Causes of LAD include:

- Normal variation (physiologic, often age-related change)
- Left ventricular hypertrophy
- Conduction defects: left bundle branch block, left anterior fascicular block
- Inferior wall myocardial infarction
- Preexcitation syndromes (e.g., Wolff-Parkinson-White syndrome)
- Ventricular ectopic rhythms (e.g., ventricular tachycardia)
- Congenital heart disease (e.g., primum atrial septal defect, endocardial cushion defect)
- Hyperkalemia
- Emphysema
- Mechanical shift, for example with expiration or raised diaphragm (e.g., pregnancy, ascites, abdominal tumor, organomegaly)
- Pacemaker-generated rhythm or paced rhythm

Causes of RAD include:

- Normal variation (e.g., children, young adults)
- Limb-lead reversal (left- and right-arm electrodes)
- Right ventricular overload syndromes (acute or chronic)
- Right ventricular hypertrophy
- Conduction defects: left posterior fascicular block, right bundle branch block
- Lateral wall myocardial infarction
- Preexcitation syndromes (e.g., Wolff-Parkinson-White syndrome)
- Ventricular ectopic rhythms (e.g., ventricular tachycardia)
- Congenital heart disease (e.g., secundum atrial septal defect)
- Dextrocardia
- Left pneumothorax
- Mechanical shift, for example with inspiration or emphysema
- Conditions that cause right ventricular strain (e.g., pulmonary embolism, pulmonary stenosis, pulmonary hypertension, chronic lung disease, and resulting cor pulmonale)

CHAPTER 8:
P-wave:

On EKG, P-wave represents Atrial depolarization.

The height of P-wave is due to RIGHT ATRIAL CONTRACTION, while the width of P-wave is because of LEFT ATRIAL CONTRACTION.

The normal amplitude of P-wave is 2.5mm (2-2.5 small squares on the y-axis)

The normal width of P-wave is 0.10 sec (2-3 small squares along the x-axis)

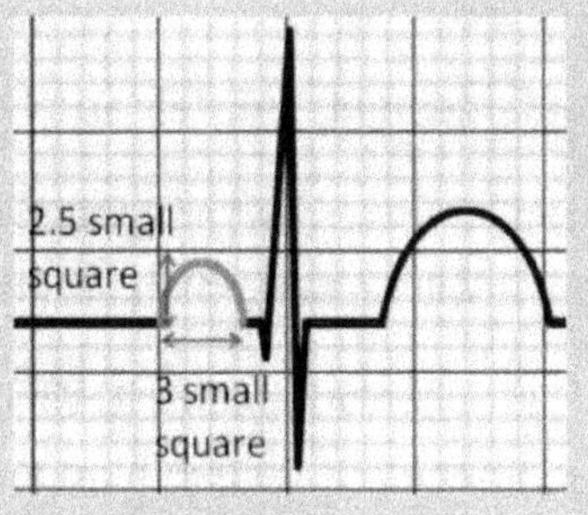

Normal P- wave
3 small square wide, and 2.5 small square high.
Always positive in lead I and II in NSR
Always negative in lead aVR in NSR
Commonly biphasic in lead V1

P-wave is always positive in the lead II, III,aVF and negative in V1

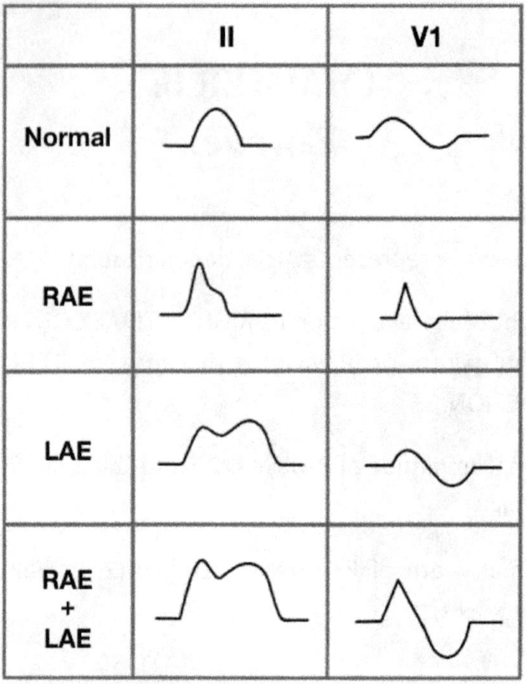

RAE=right atrial enlargement, LAE=left atrial enlargement

In case of right atrial enlargement amplitude of P-wave will be more than 2.5mm, it will be taller than normal.

In the case of left atrial enlargement, it will be broader >0.11 sec, and it will be notched or double-humped. There will be -ve deflection in lead V1.

P-waves are <u>absent in case of atrial fibrillation.</u>

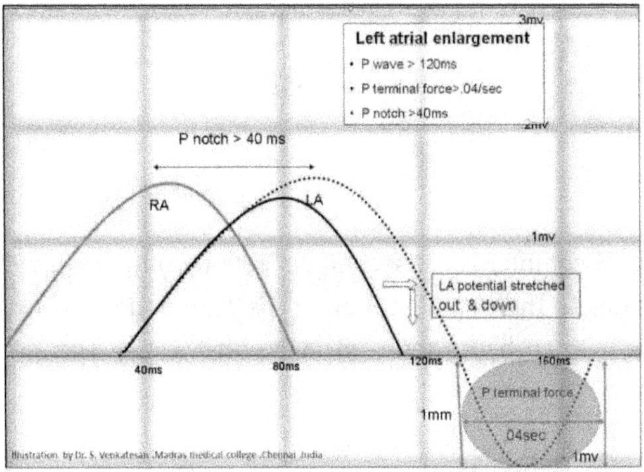
3mv
Left atrial enlargement
• P wave > 120ms
• P terminal force>.04/sec
• P notch >40ms
P notch > 40 ms
RA
LA
1mv
LA potential stretched
out & down
40ms
80ms
120ms
160ms
P terminal force
1mm
.04sec
1mv
Illustration by Dr. S. Venkatesan ,Madras medical college ,Chennai ,India

CHAPTER 9:
QRS-complex

The QRS complex is the second deflection on the regular EKG. It relates to the depolarization of the right and left ventricles of the human heart and contraction of the large ventricular muscles.

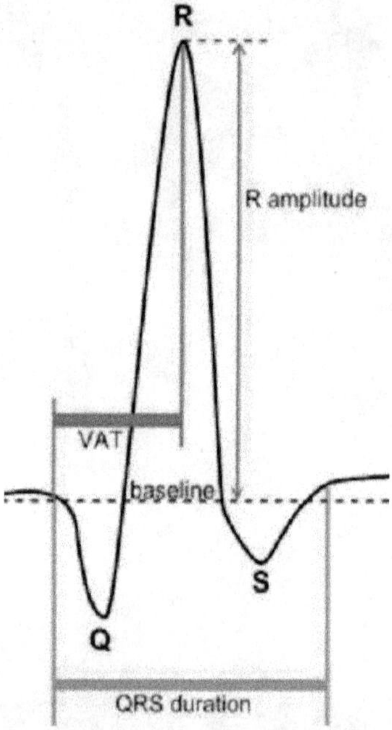

The QRS complex consists of a Q-wave, an R-wave, and S-wave, which maybe or maybe not evident, appearing either singly or in any combination. Although the complex is called the QRS complex, it does not always include a Q-wave, an R-wave, and an S-wave.

In case if the first wave of the complex is a downward deflection, the complex is considered to have a Q-wave. The next rising wave is called an R wave.

But If the first wave of the QRS is directed upward, then this wave is called an R wave. The descending wave that follows is an S wave.

Here is the nomenclature of different QRS complexes in EKG.

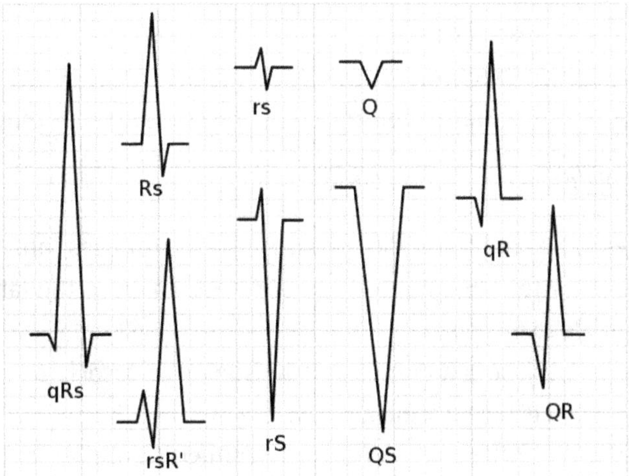

In adults, the QRS complex lasts typically **0.06–0.10 s,** this is represented by three small squares or less at the standard speed of 25 mm/s of ECG paper.

Narrow complexes (QRS < 100 ms) are usually supraventricular in origin. Broad complexes (QRS > 100 ms) are either ventricular in origin or due to abnormal conduction

Wide QRS complex:

- If QRS duration > 100 ms, it is abnormal
- A QRS duration > 120 ms is essential for the diagnosis of bundle branch block or ventricular rhythm

Following are a few reasons of broad base QRS complexes

- Bundle branch block (RBBB or LBBB)
- Hyperkalaemia
- Poisoning with sodium-channel blocking agents (e.g., the tricyclic antidepressants)
- Pre-excitation (i.e., Wolff-Parkinson-White syndrome)
- Ventricular pacing
- Hypothermia
- Intermittent aberrancy (e.g., rate-related aberrancy)

Specific patterns of wide QRS:

- The right bundle branch block produces an RSR' pattern in V1 and deep slurred S waves in the lateral leads.
- Tricyclic antidepressant poisoning is associated with sinus tachycardia and tall R' wave in aVR
- Wolff-Parkinson White syndrome is characterized by a short PR interval and delta waves
- Raised serum potassium levels (Hyperkalaemia)can present with a wide range of abnormalities including peaked T waves
- Ventricular pacing will usually have evident pacing spikes

- Hypothermia is associated with bradycardia, prolonged QT interval, Osborn waves, and shivering artifact
- In the lateral leads, left bundle branch block forms a dominant S wave in V1 with broad, notched R waves and absent Q waves

Narrow QRS complex:

Narrow (supraventricular) complexes arise from three main sites:

- Sino-atrial node (= normal P wave)
- Atria (= abnormal P wave / fibrillatory wave/ flutter wave)
- AV node/junction (= either no P wave or atypical P wave with a PR interval < 120 ms)

Right ventricular hypertrophy:

Diagnostic criteria

- If the Right axis deviation is of +110° or more.
- There is a Dominant R wave in V1 (> 7mm tall or R/S ratio > 1).
- There is a Dominant S wave in V5 or V6 (> 7mm deep or R/S ratio < 1).
- QRS duration < 120ms or 0.12sec

Causes

- Pulmonary hypertension
- Mitral stenosis
- Pulmonary embolism

- Chronic lung disease (cor pulmonale)
- Congenital heart disease like TOF
- Arrhythmogenic right ventricular cardiomyopathy

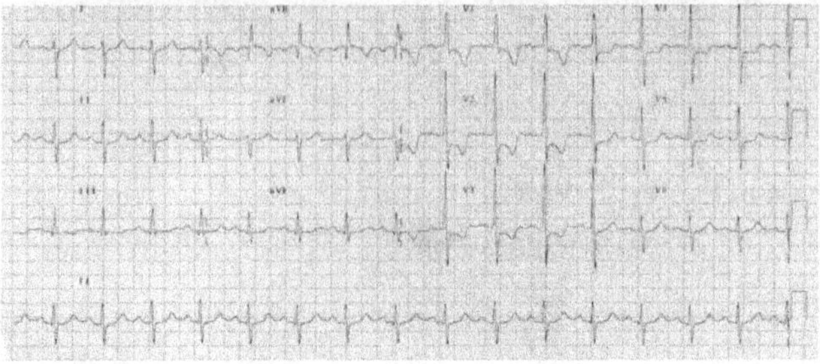

Left ventricular hypertrophy:

Diagnostic criteria:

- R wave duration in V4, V5 or V6 > 26 mm
- R wave duration in V5 or V6 plus S wave in V1 > 35 mm
- If Largest R wave plus largest S wave in precordial leads > 45 mm

Causes:

- Hypertension (most common cause)
- Aortic stenosis
- Aortic regurgitation
- Mitral regurgitation
- Coarctation of the aorta
- Hypertrophic cardiomyopathy

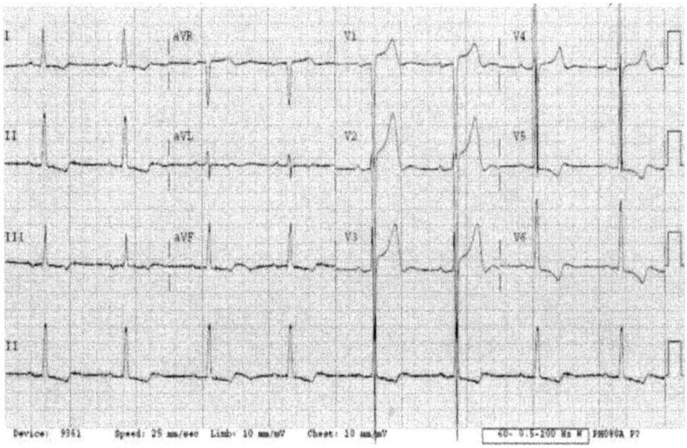

Right bundle branch blocks:

Diagnostic Criteria

- Broad QRS complex of > 120 ms
- RSR' pattern in Lead V1-3 ('M-shaped' QRS complex)
- Presence of Wide slurred S wave in the lateral leads (I, aVL, V5-6)

Causes:

- Right ventricular hypertrophy/cor pulmonale
- Pulmonary embolus
- Ischaemic heart disease
- Rheumatic heart disease
- Myocarditis or cardiomyopathy
- Degenerative disease of the conduction system
- Congenital heart disease (e.g., atrial septal defect)

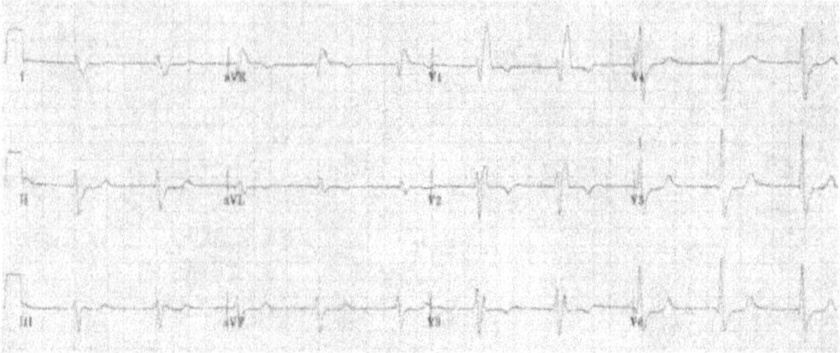

Left bundle branch block:

Diagnostic criteria:

- duration of QRS complex is > 120 ms
- Dominant S wave in V1
- Presence of Broad monophasic R wave in lateral leads (I, aVL, V5-V6)
- Absence of Q waves in lateral leads (I, V5-V6, small Q waves are still acceptable in aVL)
- Prolonged R wave with peak time > 60ms in left precordial leads (V5-6)

Causes of Left Bundle Branch Block:

- Aortic stenosis
- Ischaemic heart disease
- Hypertension
- Dilated cardiomyopathy
- Anterior MI
- League disease in which there is degeneration (fibrosis) of the conducting system
- Hyperkalaemia
- Digoxin toxicity

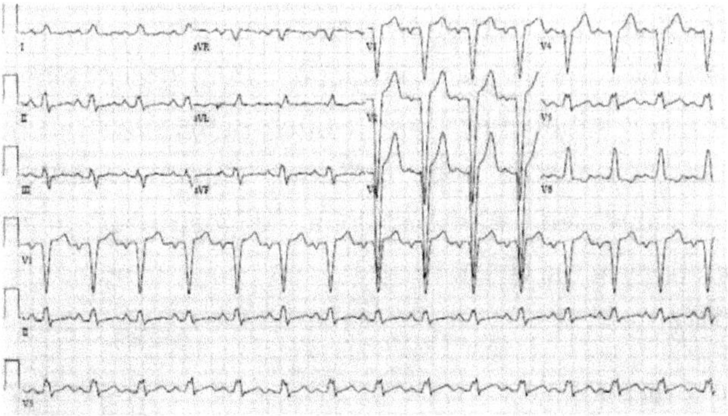

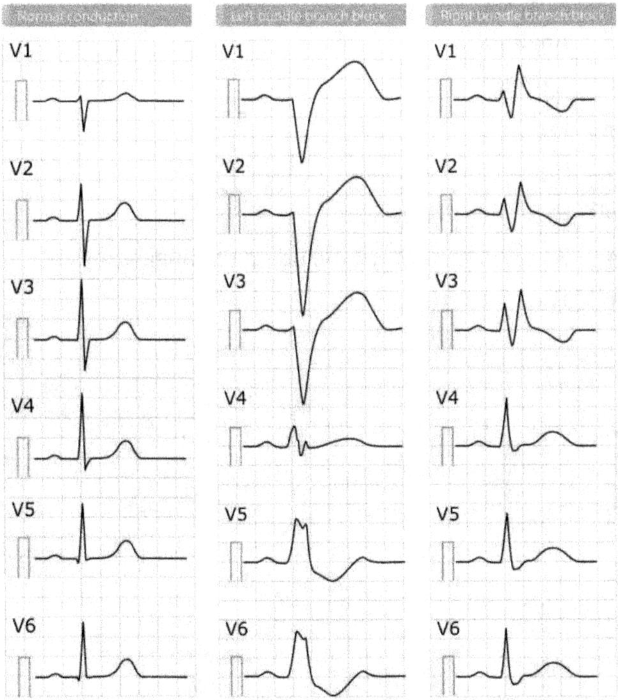

Paperspeed 50 mm/s.

Premature Ventricular contractions:

A premature ventricular contraction (PVC) occurs when the heartbeat is initiated by Purkinje fibers in the ventricles rather than by the sinoatrial node. PVCs may cause no symptoms or can be expressed as an occasional "skipped beat" or felt as palpitations in the chest. Usually, it's a benign condition. Some major causes are

- Alcohol
- Anemia
- Anxiety
- Caffeine
- Exercise
- Heart disease
- High blood pressure
- Some medications, including decongestants
- Tobacco

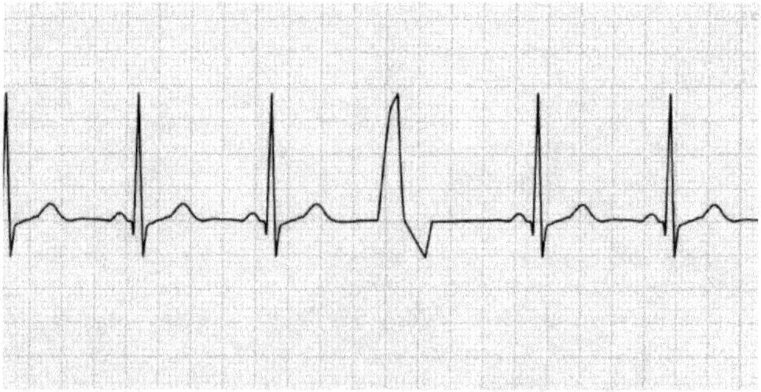

CHAPTER 10:
T-waves:

T wave represents the repolarization of the ventricle. The shape of the T wave is usually distorted with a rounded peak.

Characteristics of the normal T wave

- Upright in all leads apart from aVR, aVL, III, and V1 leads
- The amplitude of T-wave < 5mm in limb leads, < 15mm in precordial leads

T wave abnormalities

- Peaked T waves
- Hyperacute T waves
- Inverted T waves
- Biphasic T waves
- 'Camel Hump' T waves
- Flattened T waves

Flattened T waves

Flat T waves are a non-specific finding but may signify

- ischemia (if dynamic or in contiguous leads) or
- electrolyte abnormality, e.g., hypokalaemia (if generalized).

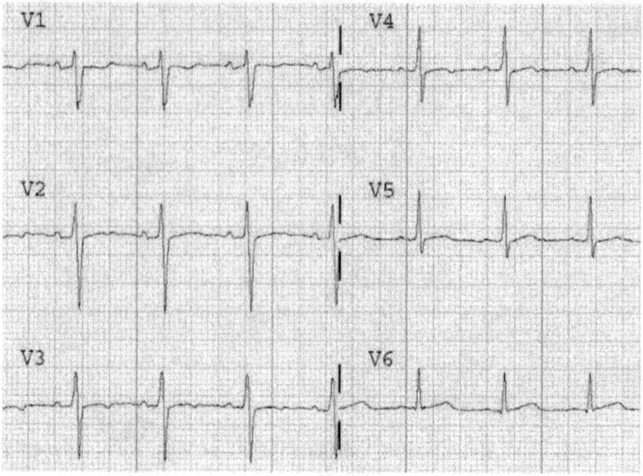

'Camel hump' T waves

It is described as T-waves that have a double peak. There are two leading causes of camel hump T waves:

- Prominent U waves fused with the T wave, as seen in severe hypokalaemia
- Hidden P waves implanted in the T wave, as seen in sinus tachycardia and various types of heart block.

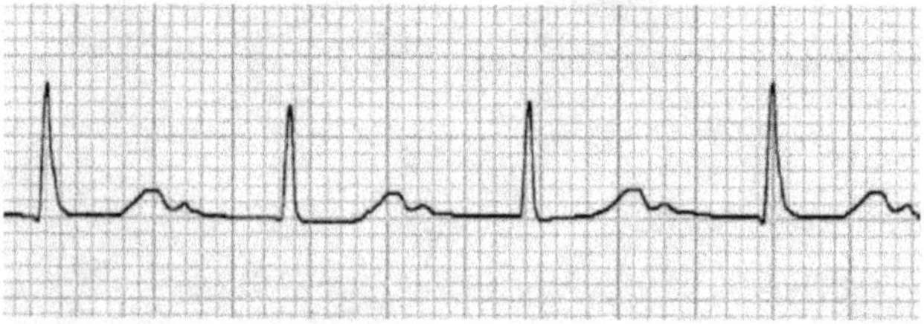

Biphasic T waves:

There are two main reasons for biphasic T waves:

- Myocardial ischemia
- Hypokalaemia

The two waves go in opposite directions:

Biphasic T waves in case of ischemia – T waves go UP then DOWN

Biphasic T waves in case of Hypokalaemia – T waves go DOWN then UP

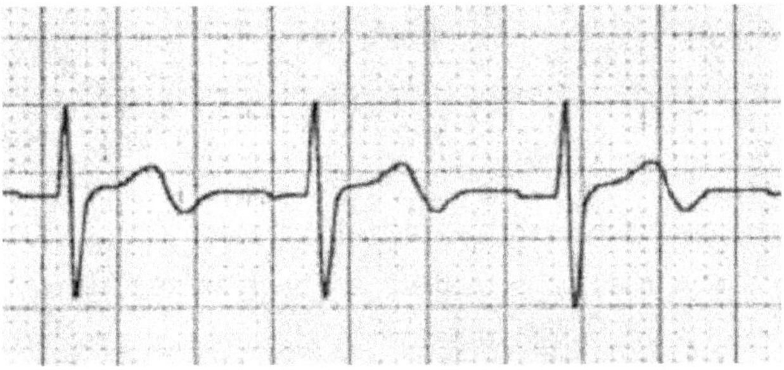

Inverted T waves:

T-wave inversion is seen in the following conditions:

- Normal finding in children
- Persistent juvenile T wave pattern
- Myocardial ischemia and infarction
- Bundle branch block
- Ventricular hypertrophy ('strain' patterns)
- Pulmonary embolism
- Hypertrophic cardiomyopathy
- Raised intracranial pressure

Inverted T-waves in lead III is a natural variant.

New T-wave inversion (compared with previous ECGs) is always abnormal.

Pathological T wave inversion is usually regular and deep (>3mm).

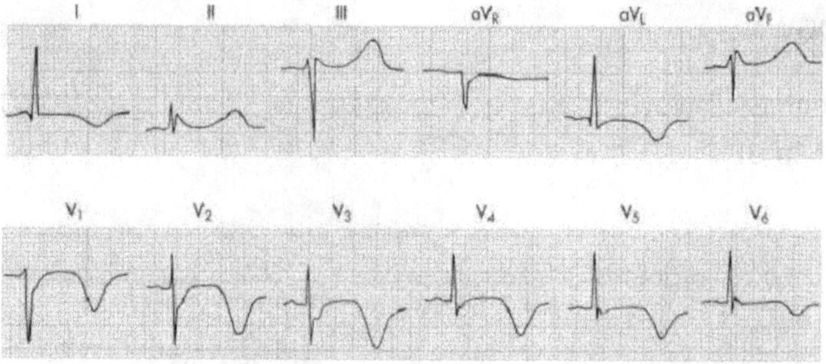

Hyperacute T waves:

Broad, asymmetrically peaked, or 'hyperacute' T-waves are observed in the early stages of ST-elevation MI (STEMI) and often precede the appearance of ST-elevation and Q waves. They are also seen with Prinzmetal angina.

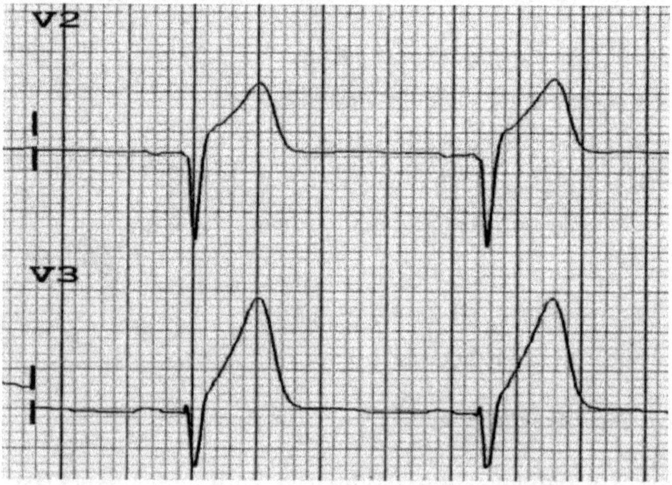

ECG Peaked T waves:

Tall, narrow, evenly peaked T-waves are characteristically seen in hyperkalemia.

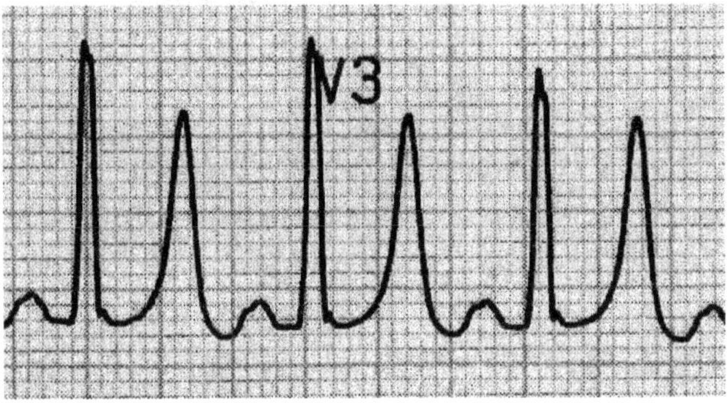

CHAPTER 11:
U-waves and Q-waves

U-waves:

The 'U' wave is a wave, which comes after the T wave of ventricular repolarization and may not always be noticed as a result of its small size. 'U' waves are thought to represent repolarization of the Purkinje fibers, but the exact source of the U wave is not clear.

Prominent U waves are most frequently seen in hypokalemia but may be present in hypercalcemia, thyrotoxicosis, congenital long QT syndrome, or exposure to digitalis, epinephrine, and Class 1A and 3 antiarrhythmics, as well as in, and in the presence of intracranial hemorrhage.

An inverted U wave may signify myocardial ischemia and left ventricular volume overload.

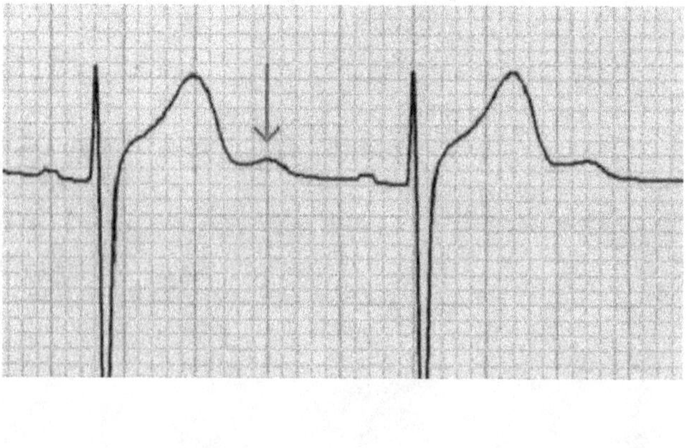

Q-waves:

- Small Q waves are considered normal in most leads
- Deeper Q waves (>2 mm) are present in leads III and lead aVR as a normal variation
- Under normal circumstances, Q waves are not present in the right-sided leads such as V1-3

Pathological Q Waves

Q waves are considered pathological if:

  - 40 ms (1 mm) wide
  - 2 mm deep
  - More than 25% of the depth of QRS complex
- Seen in leads V1-3
- Pathological Q waves usually indicate abnormal conduction of current due to prior myocardial infarction. As after MI dead part of the myocardium is replaced by scar tissue which can't conduct an electrical impulse,

Differential Diagnosis

- Myocardial infarction
- Cardiomyopathies — Hypertrophic (HOCM), infiltrative myocardial disease.
- Lead placement errors — for example, upper limb leads placed on lower limbs
- Extreme clockwise or anti-clockwise rotation of the heart

Loss of regular Q waves

- The absence of small septal Q waves in leads V5-6 should be considered as abnormal.
- The absence of Q waves in V5-6 is most commonly due to LBBB.

CHAPTER 12:
EKG segments

ST-segment:

The **ST segment** is the flat, isoelectric part of the ECG between the end of the S wave or starts at the J point (junction between the QRS complex and ST segment) and ends at the start of the T-wave. Its duration is 80 ms. It should be necessarily at level with the PR and TP segments.

The ST Segment represents the period between ventricular depolarization and repolarization.

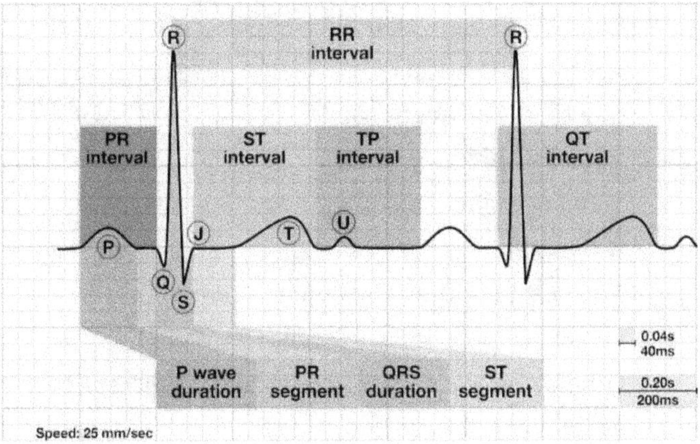

Causes of ST-Segment Elevation

An elevation of >1mm and longer than 80 milliseconds following the J-point is defined as ST-segment elevation.

- Acute myocardial infarction
- Coronary vasospasm (Printzmetal's angina)
- Pericarditis
- Benign early repolarization
- Left bundle branch block
- Left ventricular hypertrophy
- Ventricular aneurysm
- Brugada syndrome
- Ventricular paced rhythm
- Raised intracranial pressure
- Takotsubo Cardiomyopathy

Less Common Causes of ST-segment Elevation

- Pulmonary embolism and acute cor pulmonale (typically seen in lead III)
- Acute aortic dissection (usually causes inferior STEMI due to RCA dissection)
- Hyperkalaemia
- Sodium-channel blocking drugs (due to QRS widening)
- J-waves (hypothermia, hypercalcemia)
- Following electrical cardioversion
- Others: Cardiac tumor, myocarditis, pancreas or gallbladder disease

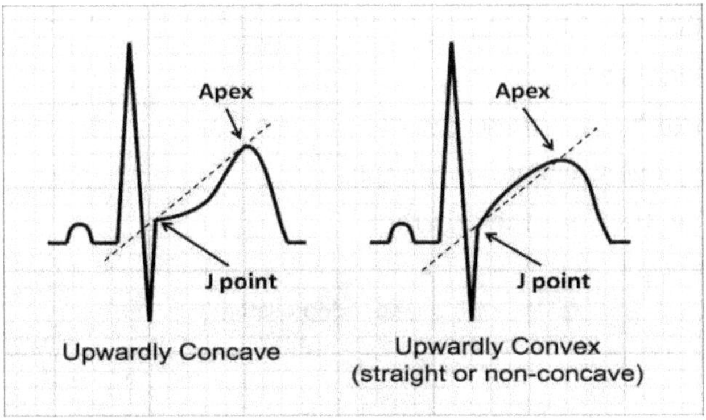

Various shapes of ST-elevation on EKG

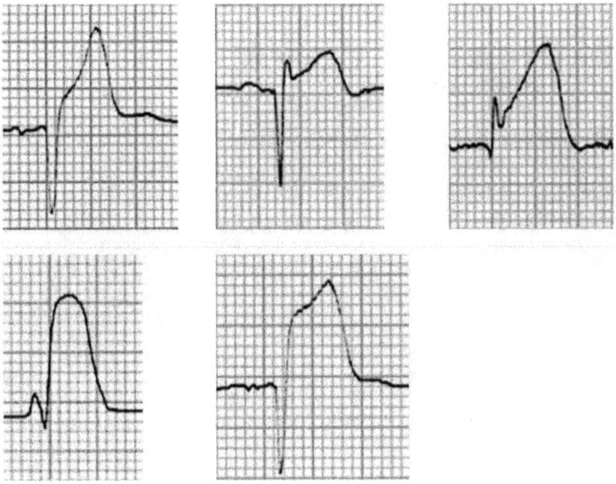

Causes of ST Depression

- Myocardial ischemia / NSTEMI
- Reciprocal change in STEMI Posterior MI
- Digoxin effect
- Hypokalaemia
- Supraventricular tachycardia

- Right bundle branch block
- Right ventricular hypertrophy
- Left bundle branch block
- Left ventricular hypertrophy
- Ventricular paced rhythm

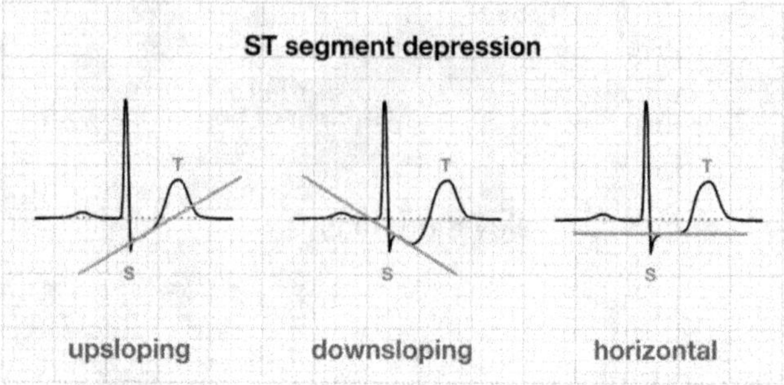

CHAPTER 13:
EKG intervals

PR Interval:

The **PR interval** is the time duration from the start of the P wave to the beginning of the QRS complex. It signifies conduction through the AV node.

- The average PR interval is between 120 – 200 ms (three to five small squares).
- If the PR interval is > 200 ms, it is labeled as a first-degree heart block.
- PR interval < 120 ms indicates pre-excitation (the presence of an accessory pathway in between the atria and ventricles) or **AV nodal (junctional) rhythm**.

1st-degree heart blocks:

The most common triggers of first-degree heart block are

- an AV nodal disease
- enhanced vagal tone (such as in athletes)
- myocarditis
- acute myocardial infarction (especially acute inferior MI)
- electrolyte disturbances
- medication (that increases the refractory time of the AV node, thereby slowing AV conduction). The group of drugs

includes <u>calcium channel blockers, beta-blockers, cardiac glycosides.</u>

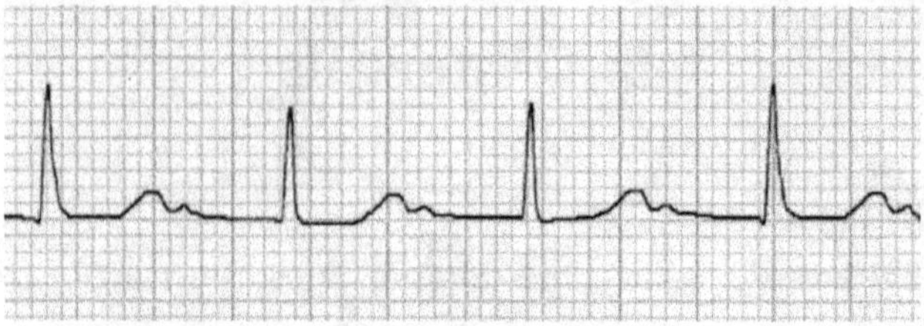

2nd-degree heart blocks:

- Second-degree heart block, Mobitz type I also known as Wenckebach phenomenon.
- The baseline PR interval is prolonged, and then further prolongs with each consecutive beat, until a QRS complex is dropped.
- The PR interval before the dropped beat is the longest, while the PR interval after the dropped beat is the shortest.

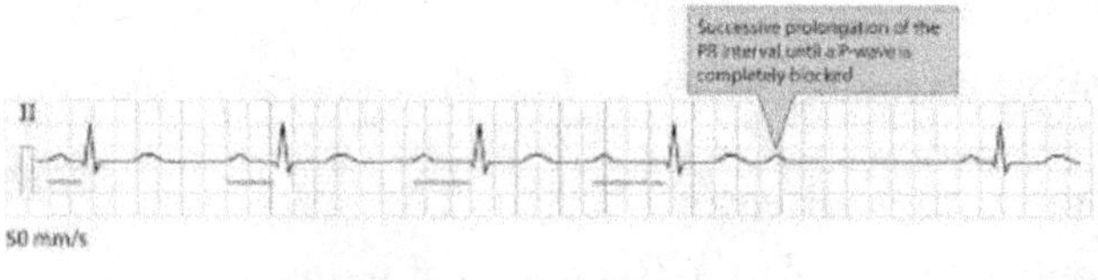

3rd-degree heart block:

In complete heart block, there is a complete lack of AV conduction – *none* of the supraventricular impulses are conducted to the ventricles.

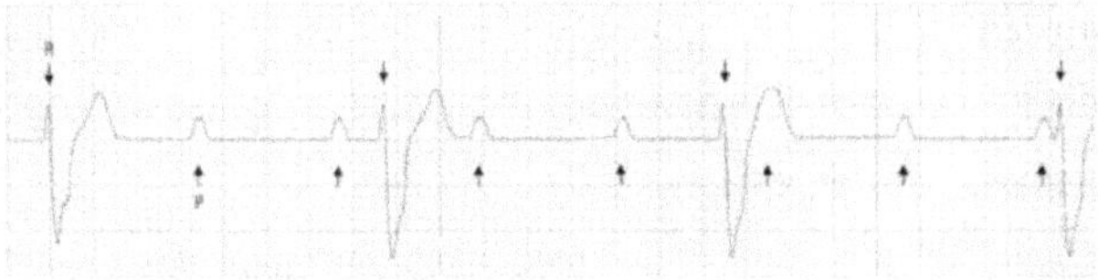

the two rates are different and independent; there is no evidence that any of the atrial impulses are conducted to the ventricles.

Causes of heart block:

- Inferior myocardial infarction
- AV-nodal blocking drugs (e.g., calcium-channel blockers, beta-blockers, digoxin)
- Idiopathic degeneration of the conducting system known as Lenegre's or Lev's disease

Heart block poem:

If the R is away from P, then you have a First Degree.

Longer, longer, longer, drop! Then you have a Wenkebach.

If some P's don't get through, then you have Mobitz II.

If P's and Q's don't agree, then you have the Third Degree

Q-T Interval:

From the starting point of the Q wave to the endpoint of the T wave on ECG paper is defined as the QT interval. It represents the duration for ventricular depolarization and repolarization.

The QT interval is most measured in the lead II, leads I and V5

An abnormally long or atypically short QT interval is associated with an increased risk of developing irregular heart rhythms and sudden cardiac death.

When the heart is rate is fast, the QT interval will become short, showing QT interval is dependent on the heart rate. So, there is a need to adjust the QT interval to improve the detection of patients at increased risk of ventricular arrhythmia.

The most used QT correction formula is the **Bazett's formula**

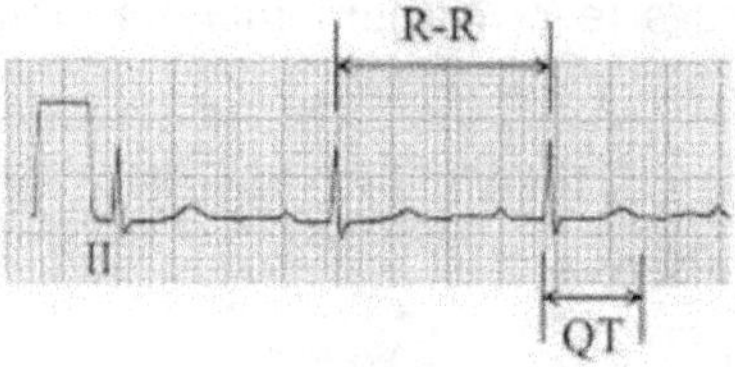

$$QTc = \frac{QT}{\sqrt{R\text{-}R}}$$

Where QTcB is the QT interval corrected for heart rate, and RR is the interval from the start of one QRS complex to the beginning of the next QRS complex.

- QTc is prolonged if its duration is > 440ms in men or > 460ms in women
- If QTc > 500 ms, it is associated with increased risk of torsades de pointes
- QTc is abnormally short if its duration is < 350ms

Causes of prolong QTc:

- Hypokalaemia
- Hypomagnesaemia
- Hypocalcemia

- Hypothermia
- Myocardial ischemia
- ROSC Post-cardiac arrest
- Raised intracranial pressure
- Congenital long QT syndrome
- Medications/Drugs

Causes of a short QTc:

- Hypercalcemia
- Congenital short QT syndrome
- Digoxin effect

R-R Interval:

RR interval, the time intervened between two successive R-waves of the QRS signal on the electrocardiogram. It is also used to calculate heart rate. Normal RR interval is 0.6-1.2 seconds

(Heart rate is a function of intrinsic properties of the sinus node as well as autonomic influences)

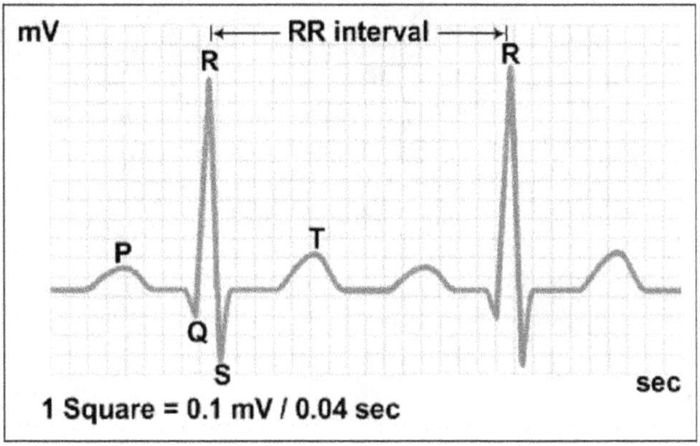

Summary:

Normal values for waves and intervals can be summarized as follows:

- RR interval: 0.6-1.2 seconds
- P wave: 80 milliseconds
- PR interval: 120-200 milliseconds
- PR segment: 50-120 milliseconds
- QRS complex: 80-100 milliseconds
- ST-segment: 80-120 milliseconds
- T wave: 160 milliseconds
- ST interval: 320 milliseconds
- QT interval: 420 milliseconds or less if the heart rate is 60 beats per minute (bpm)

Possible ECG features of healthy athletes

Variations in rhythm

- Sinus bradycardia
- Junctional rhythm
- 'Wandering' atrial pacemaker
- First-degree block
- Mobitz type 1 (Wenckebach) second-degree block

Other variations in the ECG

- Tall P waves and QRS complexes
- Prominent septal Q waves
- Counterclockwise rotation
- Tall symmetrical T waves
- Biphasic T waves
- T wave inversion in the lateral leads
- Prominent U waves

Possible ECG features of Pediatric population

At birth, the right ventricle is more abundant and thicker than the left ventricle, reflecting the higher physiological stresses placed upon it *in utero* (i.e., pumping blood through the relatively high-resistance pulmonary circulation)

Conduction intervals (PR interval, QRS duration) are much shorter than adults due to the smaller cardiac size.

Infants and neonates have a significantly faster heart rate than adults.

Common Findings on the Paediatric ECG

The following electrocardiographic features may be *normal* for healthy infants and children:

- Heart rate >100 beats/min
- Rightward QRS axis > +90°
- "juvenile T-wave pattern"-- T wave inversions in V1-3
- Dominant R wave in V1
- RSR' pattern in V1
- Marked sinus arrhythmia
- Short PR interval (< 120ms)
- QRS duration (<80ms)

- Slightly peaked P waves < 3mm in peak is considered normal if the child is less than six months old.
- Slightly long QTc (≤ 490ms in infants ≤ six months)
- in the inferior and left precordial leads, Q-waves are seen.

FETAL ECG MONITORING

Electrocardiograph (ECG) is the most widely applied non-invasive study for cardiac activity. ECG waveform provides a considerable amount of clinical information. While it has been employed extensively in different clinical conditions, its application to the intra-uterus fetus is still limited. This limitation of knowledge is mainly due to the lack of a proper mechanism to measure direct fetal ECG (fECG) signal.

There are two main reasons which highlight the importance of fetal HCG detection. First, to non-invasively obtain the fetal heart rate, so that fetal distress can be predicted before-hand. Second, to analyze the fECG to make the diagnosis of different cardiac problems. However, the fECG morphological analysis is not performed frequently in clinics or hospitals.

There are two main types of fetal ECG signals. The first kind of signal is recorded directly through an electrode attached to the fetal skin. For example, during delivery, the electrode is attached to the scalp while the cervix dilates. This is an invasive procedure that records the signal of high quality. Still, it can only be done during a specific and brief period, as the instrument is not designed for long-term monitoring. The risk of infection is also high. Therefore, *direct fECG signal* is not done routinely in clinics.

The second type of signal is recorded from the abdomen of the mother with specializes sensors. These sensor is attached close to the fetus so that the strong fECG signal could be recorded. The signal thus obtained is called the *abdominal ECG* (aECG), which is composed of both the maternal cardiac activity, (*maternal abdominal ECG (maECG)*, and the fetal cardiac activity, (*indirect fECG signal* or non-invasive fECG signal)

The aECG signal is non-invasive, easy-to-collect, and suitable for monitoring for a longer duration of time, but the fECG signal always gets mixed with the maECG.It is challenging to get standardized recording due to individual variabilities, and it is tough to interpret fetal ECG waveform due to the mingling of maternal ECG.

Different algorithms have been developed so far to overcome this problem. Various devices have been invented so far, to monitor fetal heartbeat even by using cell pho

PORTION 3:

CLINICAL CONDITIONS THAT AFFECT EKG

CHAPTER 14:
EKG changes in Acute coronary syndrome

Acute coronary syndrome (ACS) is a broad term for acute presentations of ischaemic heart disease.

The acute presentation includes the following clinical presentations,

- ST-elevation myocardial infarction (STEMI)
- non-ST elevation myocardial infarction (NSTEMI)
- unstable angina

" Ischaemia " refers to an insufficient volume of blood, and Ischemic heart disease occurs when blood supply to heart muscles gets compromised.

Ischaemic heart disease is also known as coronary heart disease and coronary artery disease.

Main reason Coronary arteries gets a block, is by a gradual build-up of fatty plaques within the walls

RISK FACTORS FOR ACUTE CORONARY SYNDROME:

Unmodifiable risk factors	Modifiable risk factors
Increasing age	Smoking
Male gender	Diabetes mellitus
Family history	Hypertension
	Hypercholesterolaemia
	Obesity

PATHOPHYSIOLOGY:

Typical structure of the blood vessel consists of the following layers

1.The intima, the innermost layer lined by a smooth tissue called endothelium

2.The media, a layer of smooth muscle

3.The adventitia, connective tissue anchoring arteries to adjacent structures

- Initial endothelial dysfunction is triggered by several risk factors such as smoking
- These factors lead to inflammatory changes in the endothelium of the artery
- Low-density lipoprotein (LDL) particles infiltrate into the subendothelial space

- Monocytes cells migrate from the blood into the subendothelial space of the vessel wall where they differentiate into macrophages.
- These macrophages then phagocytose oxidized LDL, slowly turning into large 'foam cells'.
- As these macrophages die, there is further propagation of the inflammatory process.
- Accumulation of foam cells and lipid leads to 'fatty streak formation,' which further leads to fatty plaque formation.
- Smooth muscle proliferation and migration from the media into the intima results in the formation of a fibrous capsule covering the fatty plaque leading to ATHEROMA formation.
- The atheroma results in narrowing of vessel lumen as well as hardening of the vessel wall, a condition known as Atherosclerosis

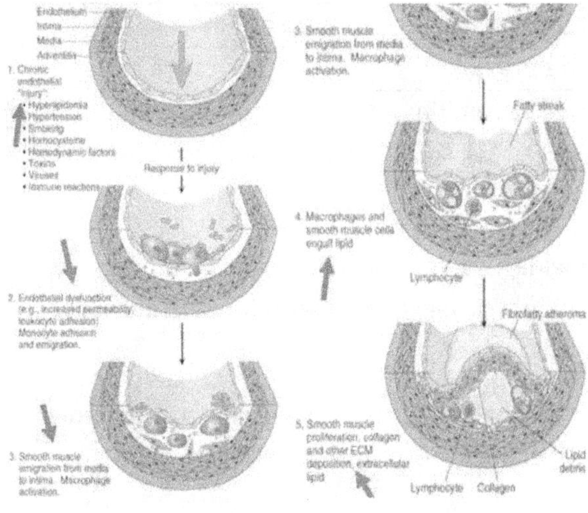

COMPLICATIONS OF ATHEROSCLEROSIS:

Once a plaque has formed, several complications can develop:

Physical blockage in the lumen of the coronary artery.Which leads to reduced blood flow to heart muscles. Particularly at times of increased demand, resulting in clinical angina. If the plaque occlude the coronary artery entirely, this may present as a myocardial infarction

ANGINA	MYOCARDIAL INFARCTION
Reduced blood supply to myocardial cells	No blood supply to myocardial cells
Aggravates by exercise or emotions	No obvious precipitant
Relieved by rest and nitrates	Not relieved by rest or nitrates
Affected myocardial cells are weakened	Affected myocardial cells die
No scar formation	Scar formation
Symptoms are mild	Symptoms are severe
No nausea or vomiting	Nausea and vomiting present
Symptoms usually last for 3-8 minutes	Symptoms are persistent

Stable angina is a feeling of discomfort or chest pain that occurs with physical activity due to interrupted supply to the heart.

Unstable angina is a condition in which myocardial tissue doesn't get enough blood flow and oxygen, but there is still no tissue damage. There are persistent symptoms not relieved by rest or vasodilators

ST-Elevation Myocardial Infarction (**STEMI**) is a severe type of myocardial infarction in which **ST-segment elevation** is detected on the **ECG leads** according to the blocked coronary artery.

Non-ST-elevation myocardial infarction (NSTEMI) is an acute ischemic event resulting in myocyte necrosis. But initial ECG may not show any changes or might show inverted ST-segment.

SIGNS AND SYMPTOMS OF ACUTE CORONARY SYNDROME:

The classic and most common characteristic of ACS is chest pain.

- typically, central/left-sided
- may radiate to the jaw or the left arm
- often described as 'heavy' or 'dull.'
- However clinically patients may present with a wide variety of complaints such as dyspepsia
- certain patients for example diabetics or aged individuals may not experience any chest pain

Other symptoms in ACS include

- dyspnoea (breathlessness)
- sweating

- nausea and vomiting

Patients presenting with ACS often have very few physical signs to elicit

- pulse, blood pressure, temperature and oxygen saturations are often normal

- In case of complications, e.g., cardiac failure then there are several findings such as pedal edema and the patient may appear pale and clammy

Differential diagnosis of chest pain:

<u>Acute chest pain</u>

- Myocardial infarction
- Pulmonary embolism
- Pneumothorax and other pleuritic diseases
- Pericarditis
- Aortic dissection

<u>Intermittent chest pain</u>

- Angina
- Oesophageal pain
- Muscular pain
- Nonspecific pain

<u>INVESTIGATIONS:</u>

The two most important investigations are

- ECG (ST-segment elevation or depression)

• cardiac markers, e.g., troponin I and troponin T (markers of myocardial cell injury)

X-ray chest and Echocardiography has no significance in acute coronary syndrome.

EKG changes in acute coronary syndrome:

On EKG, first, try to identify an abnormality in ST-segment and T-wave:

classic changes in acute myocardial infarction

- **peaked T waves with ST-elevation**
- **the gradual loss of R wave**
- **development of pathological Q wave**

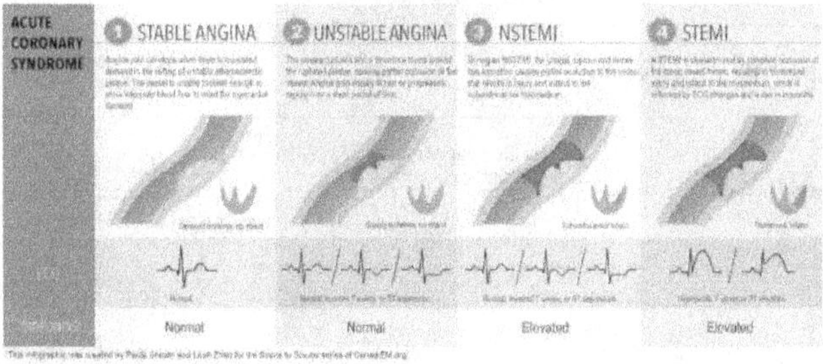

Then try to localize which leads are involved the most. It is a very crucial step as each set of leads is representing a particular surface of the heart, which in turn pointing towards the part of the heart involved.

- Septal: V1 and V2
- Anterior: V3 and V4
- Lateral: V5 and V6
- Anteroseptal: V1-V4

- Anterolateral: V3-V6
- Extensive anterior: V1-V6
- Inferior: II, III, aVF
- High Lateral: I, aVL
- Posterior: tall R wave and ST-segment depression in leads V1-V2

ECG Changes during Myocardial Infarction (MI)

Location of MI	Leads Affected	Vessel Involved	ECG Changes
Anterior wall	V_2 to V_4	• Left Anterior Descending artery (LAD) - Diagonal branch	• Poor R-wave progression • ST-segment elevation • T-wave inversion
Septal wall	V_1 and V_2	• Left Anterior Descending artery (LAD) - Septal branch	• R wave disappears • ST-segment rises • T-wave inverts
Lateral wall	I, aV_L, V_5, V_6	• Left Coronary Artery (LCA) - Circumflex branch	• ST-segment elevation
Inferior wall	II, III, aV_F	• Right coronary artery (RCA) - Posterior descending branch	• T-wave inversion • ST-segment elevation
Posterior wall	V_1 to V_4	• Left Coronary Artery (LCA) - Circumflex branch • Right Coronary Artery (RCA) - Posterior descending branch	• Tall R waves • ST-segment depression • Upright T waves

In the emergency setting, ECG is the most critical early diagnostic test for angina. It may show changes during an acute episode and in response to treatment, thus confirm a cardiac basis for clinical presentation,

Evolution of the EKG during acute myocardial infarction

	Figure	change
minutes		hyperacute T waves (peaked T waves) ST-elevation
hours		ST-elevation, with terminal negative T wave negative T wave (these can last for months)
days		Pathologic Q Waves

Pathologic Q waves are an indication of previous myocardial infarction. They are the result of the absence of electrical activity. A myocardial infarction can damage the heart muscles, and scar tissue is formed at that site. As scar tissue is electrically dead and therefore results in pathologic Q waves

The sequence of ECG changes

1. Normal ECG.

2. Raised ST segments/ tall T -waves

3. The appearance of Q waves.

4. Normalization of ST segments.

5. Inversion of T waves.

<u>Management:</u>

- prevent worsening of presenting symptoms
- revascularize (i.e. 'unblock') the vessel
- treat pain

TREAT PAIN:

for all patients with ACS

A commonly taught mnemonic for the treatment of ACS is 'MONA':

- Morphine
- Oxygen (if saturation falls below 94%)
- Nitrates
- Aspirin

REVASCULARIZATION:

For patients in which one of the coronary arteries has become occluded the priority of management is to reopen the blocked vessel

a second antiplatelet drug, e.g., clopidogrel

Thrombolysis by thrombolytic drugs

percutaneous coronary intervention (PCI (angioplasty) following which a stent may be deployed to prevent the artery occluding again

FUTURE PREVENTION:

Patients who've had an ACS need lifelong drug therapy to help reduce the risk of a further event.

- aspirin
- a second antiplatelet if suitable (e.g., clopidogrel)
- a beta-blocker
- an ACE inhibitor
- a statin

TREATMENT OPTIONS FOR NSETMI

Antithrombin treatment. Fondaparinux should be offered to patients with no identifiable risk of bleeding and who are not having angiography within the next 24 hours.or else heparin should be given Intravenous

Clopidogrel 300mg should be offered to all patients and continued for 12 months.

Glycoprotein IIb/IIIa receptor antagonists (tirofiban or eptifibatide). These are the treatment of choice for those patients who have an intermediate or increased risk of adverse cardiovascular events

Coronary angiography should be considered within four days of the initial hospital admission

Medication	Mechanism of action
Aspirin	Antiplatelet agent - inhibits the production of thromboxane A2
Clopidogrel	Antiplatelet agen- inhibits ADP binding to its platelet receptor
Enoxaparin	Activates antithrombin III, which sequentially potentiates the inhibition of coagulation factors Xa
Fondaparinux	Activates antithrombin III, which sequentially potentiates the inhibition of coagulation factors Xa
Bivalirudin	Reversible direct thrombin inhibitor

Poor prognostic factors

- age
- development (or history) of heart failure
- peripheral vascular disease
- reduced systolic blood pressure
- Killip class*
- initial serum creatinine concentration
- elevated initial cardiac markers
- cardiac arrest on admission
- ST-segment deviation

***Killip class** -This system is used to stratify risk post-myocardial infarction

Killip class	Features	30-day mortality
I	No clinical signs and symptoms of heart failure	6%
II	Lung crackles, S3	17%
III	Frank pulmonary edema	38%
IV	Cardiogenic shock	81%

COMPLICATIONS OF ACUTE CORONARY SYNDROMES

- cardiac failure
- post-infarction ischemia
- ventricular free wall rupture
    - therapy: pericardiocentesis and repair
- ventricular septal rupture

- therapy: IABP, inotropes, surgery
- acute mitral regurgitation
    - treatment: afterload reduction, IABP, inotropes, surgery ASAP
- right ventricular infarction
    - therapy: IV fluids, inotropes, AV synchrony, IABP, reperfusion
- arrhythmias
    - therapy: correct hypoxia, acidosis, hypovolaemia, K+, Mg2+ (controversial)
- cardiogenic shock
    - therapy: must get revascularization (PCI or CABG) within 24 hours
- thromboembolism
    - therapy: mural thrombus -> anticoagulant
- pericarditis and Dressler's syndrome
- complications of treatment, e.g., hemorrhage, coronary artery dissection, stent thrombosis, surgical complications.

CHAPTER 15:
EKG changes in Electrolyte imbalance

The cardiac action potential is a transitory change in membrane potential across the cell membrane of heart cells. It is due to the movement of charged atoms (called ions) between the inside and outside of the cell, through proteins known as ion channels

To appreciate the role of specific electrolyte on EKG lets review the physiology of myocardial action potential

It occurs in the bundle of His and Purkinje fibers as well

- Phase 0 = there is rapid upstroke and depolarization—voltage-gated Na+ channels open.
- Phase 1 =There is initial repolarization—inactivation of voltage-gated Na+ channels. Voltage-gated K+channels begin to open.
- Phase 2 = plateau phase—Ca2+ influx via voltage-gated Ca2+ channels balances K+ efflux. Ca2+influx triggers Ca2+ release from sarcoplasmic reticulum and contraction of myocytes.
- Phase 3 = rapid repolarization phase—massive K+ efflux due to opening of voltage-gated slow K+channels and closure of voltage-gated Ca2+ channels.
- Phase 4 = resting potential achieved again—high K+ permeability through K+ channels.

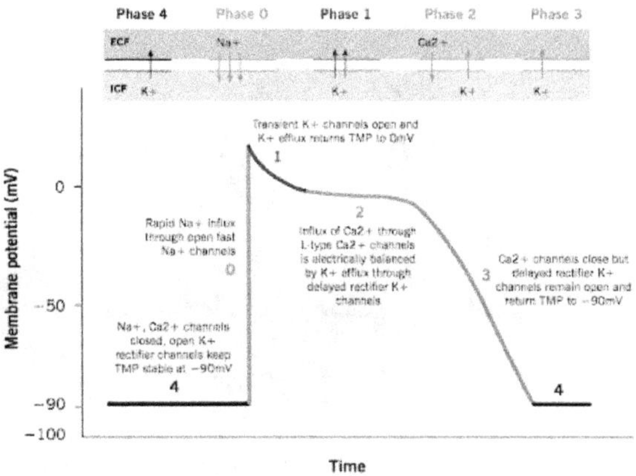

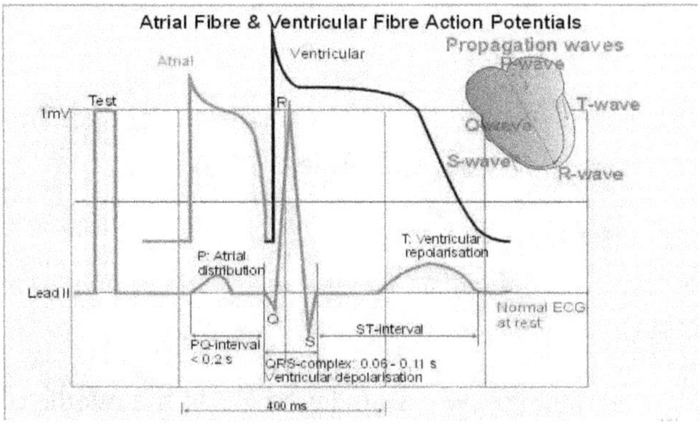

The following figure demonstrates the relation between myocardial action potential and EKG.

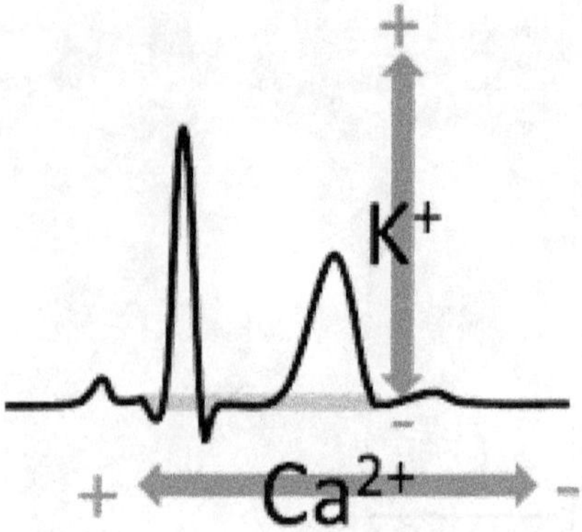

To simplify calcium ions mainly affects the QRS complex and ST-segment of EKG, while potassium ions primarily affect the amplitude and width of P and T-waves of EKG.

During electrolyte disturbance, ECG changes are generalized and not restricted to any specific lead.

Hyperkalemia:

Hyperkalemia is defined as a high level of potassium (K+) in the blood serum.

The normal range of potassium levels lies in the middle of 3.5 and 5.0 mmol/L (3.5 and 4.5 mEq/L).

- Hyperkalaemia is labeled when serum potassium level > 5.5 mEq/L
- Moderate hyperkalemia is a serum potassium > 6.0 mEq/L
- Severe hyperkalemia is a serum potassium > 7.0 mE/L

Progressive hyperkalemia leads to inhibition of impulse generation by the SA node and reduced conduction by the AV node and His-Purkinje system, subsequently resulting in bradycardia and conduction blocks and, eventually, cardiac arrest.

ECG manifestations in hyperkalemia

- Peaked T waves (TALL, TENTED T-WAVES)
- Prolonged PR segment
- Loss of P waves
- Bizarre QRS complexes (QRS complex widens)
- Sine wave

EKG findings co-relates with different potassium levels within the body:

Serum potassium > 5.5 mEq/L:

Peaked T waves (typically the earliest sign of hyperkalemia)

Serum potassium > 6.5 mEq/L:

- P wave widens and flattens
- PR segment lengthens
- P waves eventually disappear

Serum potassium > 7.0 mEq/L:

- Lengthening of QRS interval with bizarre QRS morphology
- Any conduction block like bundle branch blocks or fascicular blocks
- Sinus bradycardia or slow AF (atrial fibrillation)
- Development of a sine wave appearance (a pre-terminal rhythm)

- High-grade AV block with slow junctional rhythm and ventricular escape rhythms

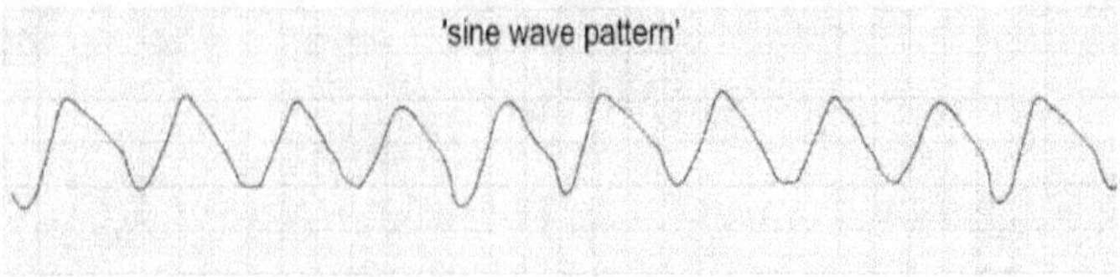

>9.0 mEq/L of Serum potassium level:

- wide, unusual complex rhythm
- Ventricular fibrillation
- Asystole

Disorders Causing Hyperkalemia

Disorders leading to hyperkalemia caused by impaired renal excretion of potassium

- Acquired hyporeninemic hypoaldosteronism
- Addison's disease
- Congenital adrenal hyperplasia (recessive or autosomal dominant)
- Mineralocorticoid deficiency
- Primary hypoaldosteronism or hyporeninemia
- Pseudohypoaldosteronism
- Renal insufficiency or failure
- Systemic lupus erythematosus
- Type IV renal tubular acidosis

<u>Disorders leading to hyperkalemia caused by a shift of potassium into the extracellular space</u>

- Acidosis
- Damage to tissue from rhabdomyolysis, burns, or trauma
- Familial hyperkalemic periodic paralysis
- Hyperosmolar states, (e.g., uncontrolled diabetes, glucose infusions)
- Insulin deficiency or resistance
- Tumor lysis syndrome

Management of Hyperkalemia:

<u>Calcium gluconate</u>

- Dosage is 10 to 20 mL of 10 percent solution IV over two to three minutes
- Onset is Immediate
- Its Effect lasts for 30 minutes
- It Protects myocardium from toxic effects of calcium but causes no effect on serum potassium level
- It Can worsen digoxin toxicity

<u>Insulin</u>

- Dosage is Regular insulin 10 units IV with 50 mL of 50 percent glucose
- Onset is within 15 to 30 minutes
- Its effect lasts for two to six hours
- It Shifts potassium from serum into the cells, but it causes no effect on total body potassium

- Consider 5 percent dextrose solution infusion at 100 mL per hour to prevent hypoglycemia in case of repeated doses of insulin. Glucose infusion should be stopped if blood sugar gets elevated above 250 mg per dL (13.9 mmol per L)

<u>Albuterol (Ventolin)</u>

- Dose:10 to 20 mg by nebulizer over 10 minutes (use the concentrated form, 5 mg per mL)
- The onset of effect:15 to 30 minutes
- The effect lasts up to two to three hours
- It Shifts potassium into the cells, become additive to the effect of insulin but no effect on total body potassium
- May cause a momentary initial rise in serum potassium

<u>Furosemide (Lasix)</u>

- Dose:20 to 40 mg IV, give with saline if volume depletion is a concern
- The onset of action:15 minutes to one hour
- Effects last for Four hours
- Increases renal excretion of potassium
- Only useful if the adequate renal response to loop diuretic

<u>Sodium polystyrene sulfonate (Kayexalate)</u>

- Dose Oral: 50 g in 30 mL of sorbitol solution Rectal: 50 g in a retention enema

- The onset of action in One to two hours (the rectal route is faster)
- The effect lasts up to four to six hours
- Removes potassium from the gut in trade for sodium
- Sorbitol may be associated with bowel necrosis. May lead to sodium retention

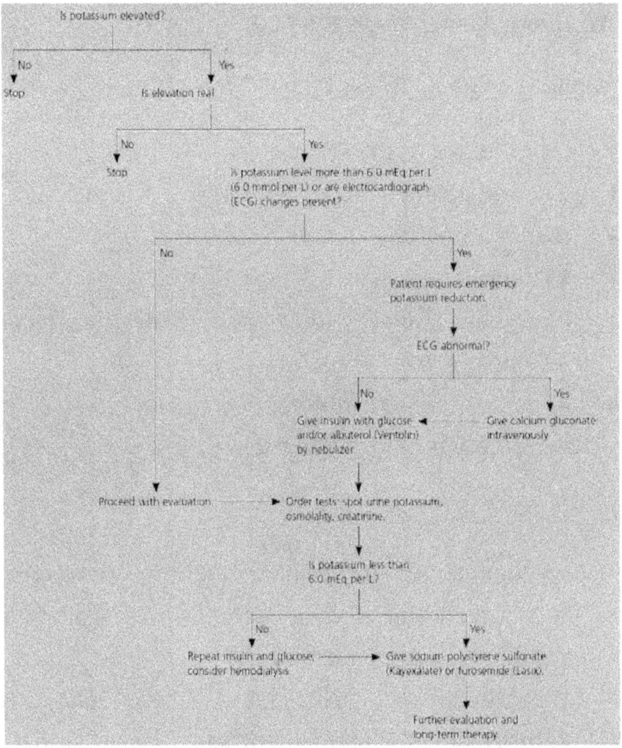

Hypokalemia

- Hypokalaemia is labeled when the level of potassium in the blood is < 3.5 mmol/L
- Moderate hypokalaemia is when the serum level of potassium is < 3.0 mmol/L
- Severe hypokalaemia is defined as a blood potassium level of < 2.5 mmol/L

Effects of hypokalaemia on the ECG

ECG changes when K+ is less than 2.7 mmol/l:

- Lengthening of the PR interval
- T wave flattening and inversion
- Higher amplitude and width of the P wave
- ST depression
- Prominent U waves (best observed in the precordial leads)
- Apparent long QT interval due to the fusion of the T and U waves (= long QU interval)

With worsening hypokalaemia:

- Frequent supraventricular and ventricular ectopics
- Supraventricular tachyarrhythmias: Atrial fibrillation, atrial flutter, atrial tachycardia
- life-threatening ventricular arrhythmias, e.g., Ventricular Fibrillation, Ventricular Tachycardia, and Torsades de Pointes can develop

Causes of hypokalemia:

Causes of potassium loss include:

- Alcohol use (excessive)
- Chronic kidney disease
- Diabetic ketoacidosis
- Diarrhea
- Diuretics (water retention relievers)
- Excessive laxative use
- Excessive sweating
- Folic acid deficiency
- Primary aldosteronism
- Some antibiotic use
- Vomiting

Occasionally, hypokalemia is caused by not getting enough potassium in the diet.

Signs and symptoms of Hypokalemia:

- weakness
- fatigue
- constipation
- muscle cramping
- palpitations

if levels fall below 2.5mmol/l

- paralysis
- respiratory failure
- breakdown of muscle tissue
- ileus (lazy bowels)

In more severe cases, abnormal rhythms may occur. It is most common in people who take digitalis medications (digoxin) or have irregular heart rhythm conditions.

Treating low potassium levels:

1. Identify Remove Or treat the cause

2. Restore potassium levels by potassium supplements.

3.Close monitoring of potassium levels at regular intervals to prevent hyperkalemia

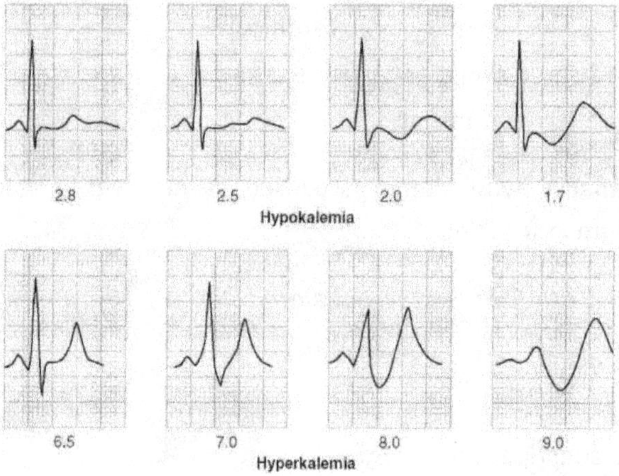

ECG Changes with Potassium Imbalance

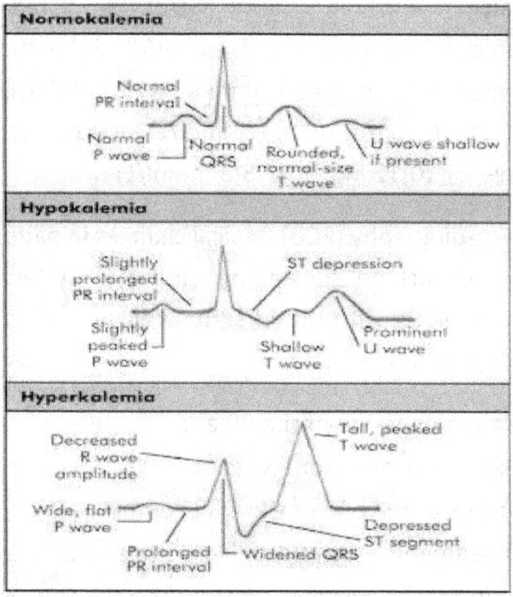

ECG EKG Changes in Hypokalemia and Hyperkalemia

Hypercalcemia

The normal level of calcium in the body is defined as,

- Total blood calcium level of 8.5 to 10.3 milligrams per deciliter (mg/dL)
- Ionized calcium levels in the blood of 4.4 to 5.4 mg/dl

Hypercalcemia may be classified based on total serum and ionized calcium levels, as following,

- Mild hypercalcemia is defined as Total Calcium level of 10.5-11.9 mg/dL (2.5-3 mmol/L) or Ionized Calcium level of 5.6-8 mg/dL (1.4-2 mmol/L)

- Moderate hypercalcemia is diagnosed as Total Calcium level of 12-13.9 mg/dL (3-3.5 mmol/L) or Ionized Calcium level of 8-10 mg/dL (2-2.5 mmol/L)
- Hypercalcemic crisis is defined as Total Calcium level of 14-16 mg/dL (3.5-4 mmol/L) or Ionized Calcium level of 10-12 mg/dL (2.5-3 mmol/L)

On electrocardiography (ECG), typical changes in patients with hypercalcemia include shortening of the QT interval. ECG changes in patients with raised serum calcium levels include the following features,

- Slight elongation of the PR and QRS intervals
- T wave flattening or inversion
- J wave at the end of the QRS-complex.
- ST-segment elevation like in acute myocardial infarction

J wave is shown by an arrow in the picture below

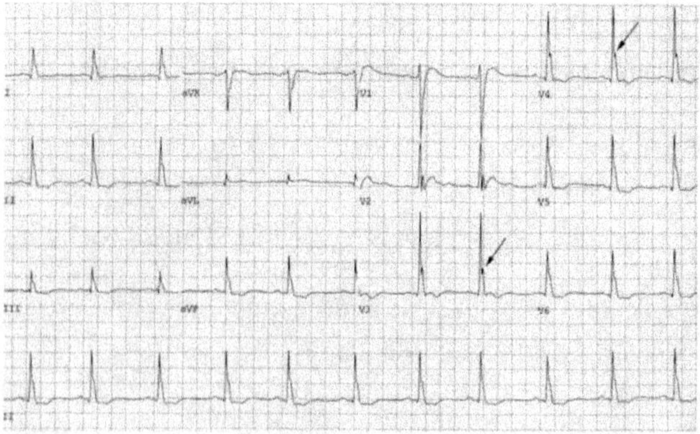

Hypercalcemia affects nearly every organ in the body. Especially It has marked effects on the central nervous system (CNS) and the kidneys. CNS effects include the following:

- Lethargy
- Weakness
- Confusion
- Coma

Renal effects include the following:

- Polyuria
- Nocturia
- Dehydration
- Renal stones
- Renal failure

Gastrointestinal effects include the following:

- Constipation
- Nausea
- Anorexia
- Pancreatitis
- Gastric ulcer

Cardiac effects include syncope from arrhythmias. Calcium has a positive inotropic effect. Hypercalcemia also causes hypertension, apparently due to renal dysfunction and direct vasoconstriction.

Treatment of hypercalcemia includes the following:

- Volume repletion with an isotonic sodium chloride solution
- Loop diuretics
- Bisphosphonates
- Peritoneal dialysis or hemodialysis
- Surgical correction of hyperparathyroidism

Hypocalcemia

Hypocalcemia is defined as a serum calcium level is < 8.8 mg/dL (< 2.20 mmol/L) or as a serum ionized calcium concentration < 4.7 mg/dL (< 1.17 mmol/L) in the presence of normal plasma protein level.

EKG changes:

- Acute hypocalcemia may clinically present as ventricular dysrhythmias as it causes prolongation of the QT interval.
- Heart failure, hypotension, and angina can also occur due to decreased myocardial contractility.

Due to the multiple cardiovascular effects, Acute hypocalcemia may clinically present as syncope, chronic heart failure (CHF), and angina.

Neuromuscular symptoms include the following:

- feelings of Numbness and tingling in the perioral area or the fingers and toes
- Muscle cramps, especially in the muscles of the back and lower extremities

- Tetany is unrelieved and forceful contractions of the hands and in the large muscles of the rest of the body commonly associated with hypocalcemia.
- Trousseau sign is a sign of latent tetany (eliciting carpal spasm by inflating the blood pressure cuff and maintaining the cuff pressure above systolic)
- Chvostek's sign of latent tetany (tapping of the inferior portion of the cheekbone will produce facial spasms)
- Brisk reflexes
- Wheezing; may develop from bronchospasm
- Dysphagia
- Voice changes (due to laryngospasm which could be fatal)

Neurologic symptoms of hypocalcemia manifest as the following symptoms:

- Irritability
- impaired intellectual capacity
- depression
- personality changes
- Fatigue
- Seizures (for example grand mal, petit mal, focal)
- Other uncontrolled movements

Chronic hypocalcemia may present as the following dermatologic manifestations:

- Coarse hair
- Brittle nails
- Psoriasis

- Dry skin
- Chronic pruritus
- Poor dentition
- Cataracts

Treatment of hypocalcemia:

- In acute cases, Intravenous calcium gluconate 10% should be given. If hypocalcemia is severe, calcium chloride could be given instead.
- In both acute or chronic conditions, maintenance doses of both calcium and vitamin-D (often as 1,25-(OH)2-D3, i.e., calcitriol) are necessary to prevent further decline.

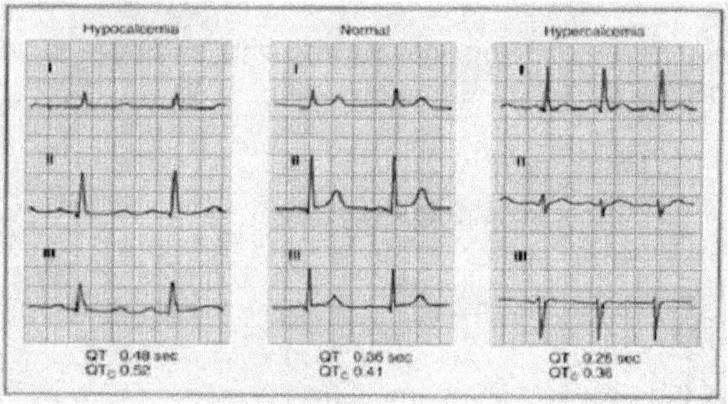

Hypomagnesemia

Magnesium acts as a physiologic **calcium blocker**, resulting in electrical conduction abnormalities within the heart.

Normal level of serum magnesium = 0.8 – 1.0 mmol/L.

Hypomagnesaemia = <0.8 mmol/L

EKG findings:

- The primary ECG abnormality seen with hypomagnesemia is a prolonged QTc.
- Atrial and ventricular ectopy
- atrial tachyarrhythmias
- torsades de pointes

Clinical signs and symptoms:

- nausea
- vomiting
- weakness
- decreased appetite

As magnesium deficiency worsens, symptoms may include:

- numbness
- tingling
- muscle cramps
- seizures
- muscle spasticity
- personality changes
- abnormal heart rhythms

Common causes of low magnesium include:

- Alcohol use
- Burns that involves a large part of the body
- Chronic diarrhea

- medical conditions causing excessive urination (polyurea) such as in uncontrolled diabetes mellitus and during recovery from acute kidney failure
- Hyperaldosteronism (a disorder in which excessive amount of the hormone aldosterone releases an into the blood from the adrenal gland)
- Kidney tubule disorders
- Malabsorption syndromes, such as celiac disease.
- Drugs including amphotericin, cisplatin, cyclosporine, proton pump inhibitors, diuretics, and aminoglycoside antibiotics
- Pancreatitis (swelling and inflammation of the pancreas)
- Excessive sweating
- Malnutrition

Treatment:

- The degree of insufficiency and clinical sign and symptoms determines the mode of Treatment for hypomagnesemia.
- For the people with mild symptoms, replacement by mouth is appropriate, whereas an intravenous drug is mandatory for people with severe effects
- Magnesium citrate has more bioavailable than oxide or amino-acid chelate forms.
- Food sources of magnesium include soybean, leafy green vegetables, nuts, fruits, and eggs

Hypermagnesemia

Hypermagnesemia is a disorder in which there is a high level of magnesium in the blood.

Diagnosis is based on a blood level of magnesium if greater than 1.1 mmol/L (2.6 mg/dL).

- mild (~2.3–4.0 mg/dL or ~0.96–1.64 mmol/L or ~1.9–3.3 mEq/L)
- moderate (~4.0–7.0 mg/dL or ~1.64–2.88 mmol/L or ~3.3–5.8 mEq/L)
- severe (>7.0 mg/dL or >2.88 mmol/L or >5.8 mEq/L).

Signs and Symptoms:

- Weakness
- Confusion
- decreased breathing rate
- decreased reflexes.
- Nausea
- Low blood pressure
- Abnormal heart rhythms and asystole
- Dizziness
- Sleepiness

Consequences related to serum concentration:

- 4.0 mEq/L decreased reflexes
- >5.0 mEq/L Prolonged atrioventricular conduction
- >10.0 mEq/L Complete heart block
- >13.0 mEq/L cardiac arrest

ECG (as for hyperkalemia)

- Increase PR and QTc
- Prolonged QRS
- Peaked T waves
- flattened p waves
- Complete AV block and asystole

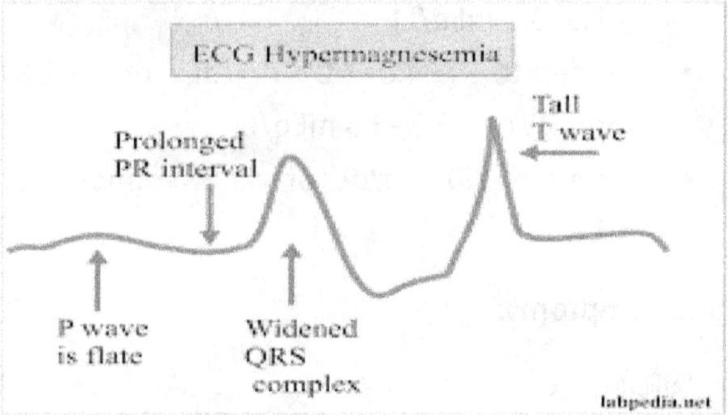

Causes of hypermagnesaemia

1) Iatrogenic
   - Hyperalimentation
   - IV and oral magnesium
   - Laxatives, enemas, antacids (especially in elderly and renal failure)
2) Renal Failure
3) Other
   - Perforated viscus with continued oral intake
   - Tumor lysis (Increased K, Mg, PO4 and decreased Ca)
   - Rhabdomyolysis

Treatment:

- Discontinue magnesium intake
- Antagonising Mg with Calcium
- Removing Magnesium from serum
- Dialysis – Treatment of choice
- Calcium chloride 10% in 5-10ml repeated
- Treats life-threatening arrhythmia
- Forced diuresis
- IV normal saline and Frusemide
- Lookout for hypocalcemia which can make symptoms worse

Insite of the fact that sodium plays a major role in the start of the action potential, its altered serum level doesn't cause a significant change on EKG unless and until serum sodium levels are very high >200mmol/l.

Electrolyte Abnormality	Electrocardiographic Findings
Hypokalemia	Decreased T wave amplitude T wave inversion ST segment depression Prominent U Wave Prolongation of QT(U) Interval Ventricular tachycardia Torsades de pointes
Hyperkalemia	
Mild	Large amplitude T waves "Peaked" or "tented" T waves
Moderate	PR interval prolongation Decreased P wave amplitude, disappearance QRS complex widening Conduction blocks with escape beats
Severe	Sine-wave pattern Ventricular fibrillation Asystole
Hypocalcemia	Prolongation of QTc interval Ventricular dysrhythmias Torsades de pointes
Hypercalcemia	Shortening of QTc interval Bradydysrhythmias
Hypo/ Hypermagnesemia	No unique electrocardiographic abnormalities, but often associated with calcium abnormalities

CHAPTER 16:
EKG changes during drug toxicities and poisonings

Poisoning is defined as exposure to any drug, chemical, or toxin that results in injury. The ECG is one of the essential tools in the assessment and management of poisoned patients for:

- screening
- diagnosis

- prognosis
- monitoring progression to guide management.

Myocardial effects of cardiotoxic drugs have particular and well-described electrocardiographic manifestations.

APPROACH TO THE ECG IN TOXICOLOGY:

- Rate and Rhythm
- PR interval –to access the degree of heart block
- Determine QRS duration in lead II in tricyclic antidepressant intoxication
- Check for Right Axis Deviation
  A massive R wave in lead aVR or increased R/S ratio indicates slow rightward conduction and is characteristic of fast sodium channel blockers.
- Determine QT interval
  Prolonged QT interval predisposes to the formation of torsade de pointe, which is more likely to occur where there is co-existing bradycardia.
- The risk of arrhythmias produced by any for drug-induced QT prolongation is accurately predicted by the "QT nomogram" In which we plot QT versus heart rate.
- Look for any Indication of increased cardiac ectopy or automaticity
- Look for Evidence of myocardial ischemia in EKG.

Sodium channels blockers:

As we have discussed previously that phase 0 of the myocardial action potential is due to Fast sodium channels.

Fast sodium channel blockade leads to slowed phase 0 of the cardiac action potential resulting in

- Widened QRS
- Right axis deviation
- Bradycardia (although tachycardia secondary to other factors is more commonly observed)
- Ventricular tachycardia and ventricular fibrillation

Examples of drugs leading to blockage of sodium channels:

- Tricyclic antidepressants
  Amitriptyline, Desipramine, Dothiepin, Imipramine, Nortriptyline
- Class 1A antidysrhythmic agents
  Disopyramide, Procainamide, Quinidine
- Class 1C antidysrhythmic agents
  Encainide, Flecainide
- Local anesthetics
  Bupivacaine, Cocaine, Ropivacaine
- Phenothiazines
  Thioridazine
- Antimalarials
  Chloroquine, Hydroxychloroquine, Quinine
- Amantadine
- Diltiazem
- Diphenhydramine
- Carbamazepine
- Propoxyphene/dextropropoxyphene
- Propranolol

Tricyclic antidepressants

Clinical Features of Tricyclic Overdose

In overdose, the tricyclics produce the following symptoms rapidly (within 1-2 hours):

- Sedation and coma
- Seizures
- Hypotension
- Tachycardia
- Broad complex dysrhythmias

ECG changes:

QRS duration of > 100 ms in lead II

- QRS duration of >100ms (2.5 small squares) is related to seizures

- QRS duration of >160ms (4 small squares) is linked with ventricular dysrhythmias

There is Right axis deviation of the terminal QRS complexes:

o Terminal R wave >3 mm in aVR

o R/S ratio >0.7 in aVR.

Patients with a tricyclic overdose will also usually demonstrate sinus tachycardia secondary to muscarinic (M1) receptor blockade.

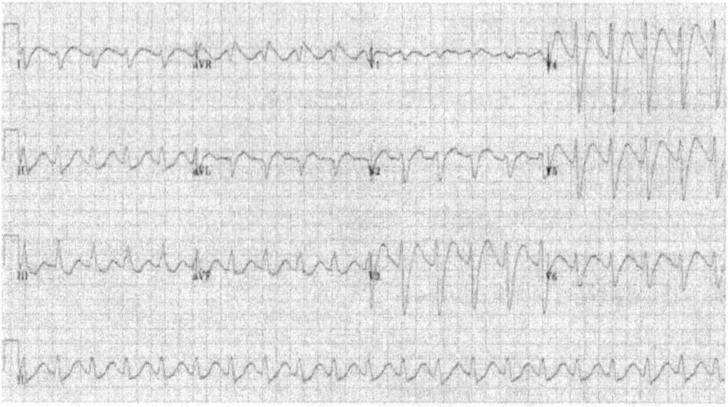

Management of TCA overdose:

Overdose of TCA is defined as the dose is taken>10mg/kg with Signs of cardiotoxicity (ECG changes)

- Patients should be managed under strict supervision and a highly equipped facility for airway management and resuscitation.
- Secure IV line, give high flow oxygen and attach monitoring equipment.
- Administer intravenous bolus of sodium bicarbonate 100 mEq (1-2 mEq/kg). The dose can be repeated after every few minutes until BP improves, and QRS complexes begin to narrow.
- Intubate as soon as possible.
- Hyperventilate to maintain a pH of 7.50 – 7.55.
- After securing the airway, place a nasogastric tube and give 50g (1g/kg) of activated charcoal.
- Treat seizures with IV benzodiazepines (e.g. diazepam 5-10mg).

- Initially, Treat hypotension with a crystalloid bolus (10-20 mL/kg). If this is unsuccessful, then consider starting vasopressors (e.g., noradrenaline infusion).
- If arrhythmias occur, the first step is to give more sodium bicarbonate then hyperventilation. Lidocaine (1.5mg/kg) IV is a third-line agent if pH is > 7.5.
- Avoid certain drugs like Ia (procainamide) and Ic (flecainide) antiarrhythmics, beta-blockers, and amiodarone because they may worsen hypotension and conduction abnormalities.
- For proper monitoring and management admit the patient to the intensive care unit

Potassium efflux blockers:

Blockade of potassium efflux during cardiac repolarization effects phase 1 and phase 3 of the myocardial action potential

ECG changes:

- Prolongation of the QT interval
- Torsade de Pointes
- T-wave abnormalities
- U-waves

Torsade de Pointes

Torsades de pointes means twisting of the points

- Polymorphic ventricular tachycardia which is characterized by shifting of sinusoidal waveforms on ECG
- It can progress to ventricular fibrillation (VF).
- Long QT interval predisposes to torsades de pointes.
- It is caused by drugs ↓ K^+, ↓ Mg^{2+}, congenital abnormalities.
- Treatment includes magnesium sulfate.

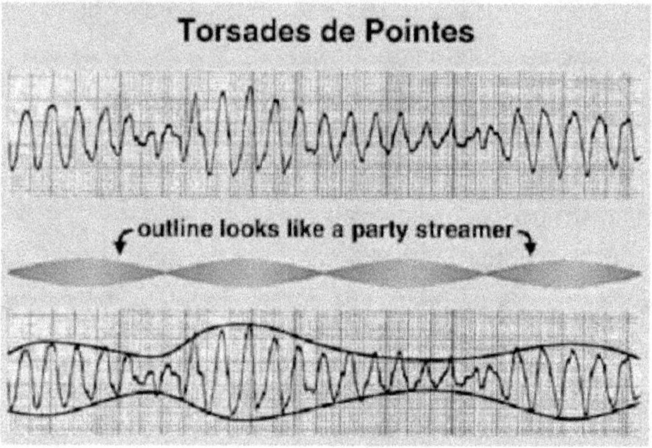

POTASSIUM EFFLUX BLOCKERS

- Antipsychotic agents
  Amisulpride, Chlorpromazine, Droperidol, Haloperidol, Quetiapine, Olanzapine, Thioridazine
- Class 1A antidysrhythmic agents
- Quinidine
- Disopyramide
- Procainamide

- Class 1C antidysrhythmic agents
  Encainide, Flecainide
- Class III antidysrhythmic agents
  Sotalol, Amiodarone
- Tricyclic antidepressants
  Amitriptyline, Desipramine, Dothiepin, Imipramine, Nortriptyline
- Other antidepressants
  Citalopram, Escitalopram, Bupropion, Moclobemide
- Antihistamines
  Diphenhydramine, Astemizole, Loratadine, Terfenadine
- Antimalarials
  Chloroquine, Hydroxychloroquine, Quinine
- Amantadine
- Macrolides
  Erythromycin

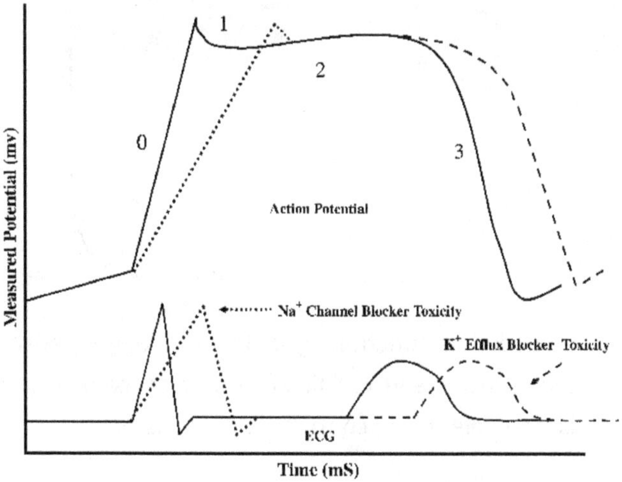

Sodium channel blocking agents mainly alters QRS complex duration and morphology while K+channels blockers prolong QT interval and produce T-wave abnormalities.

Na+-K+-ATPase pump blockade by cardiac glycosides

- Cellular Na+/K+-ATPase is an ion transport system that moves sodium ions out of the cell and brings potassium ions inside the cell.
- Due to this ion transport system cell maintains its negative membrane potential and viability of the cell.
- In Cardiac myocytes, there is a Na+-Ca++ exchanger that is essential for maintaining sodium and calcium hemostasis within the cell, along with the Na+-K+-ATPase pump.

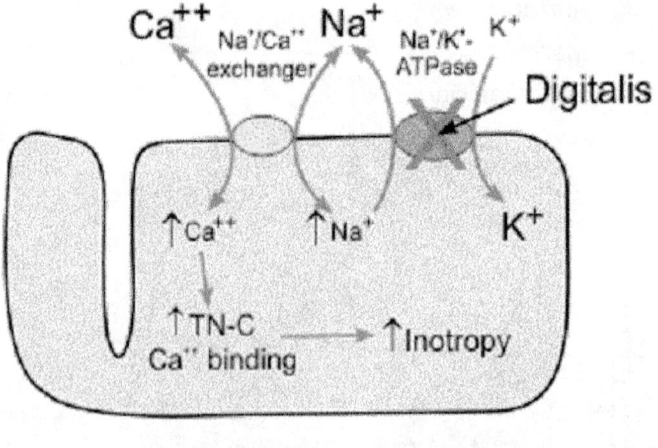

- The reverse functioning of this exchanger causes an increase in the intracellular calcium concentration that is available to the contractile proteins.

- Increased intracellular calcium prolongs Phase 4 and phase 0 of the cardiac action potential, which leads to a decrease in heart rate.
- Increased amounts of Ca2+ also leads to more storage of calcium in the sarcoplasmic reticulum. Thus causing a corresponding increase in the release of calcium during each action potential, which leads to amplified contractility (the force of contraction) of the heart without increasing heart energy expenditure.

Digoxin toxicity:

Digoxin is the cardiac glycoside which is used in the treatment of heart failure and atrial fibrillation

Signs of digoxin toxicity:

The classic features of digoxin toxicity are

- Nausea
- Vomiting
- abdominal pain
- headache
- dizziness
- confusion
- delirium
- vision disturbance (blurred or yellow vision).

cardiac disturbances include

- irregular heartbeat
- ventricular tachycardia

- ventricular fibrillation
- sinoatrial block and AV block.
- Increased automaticity
- Reduced AV node conduction (1st to 3rd-degree heart block)

EKG findings:

Keep in mind that "Drug effects" on the ECG are distinguished from "drug toxicity."

If a patient is taking digoxin, the following changes could be seen on ECG

- ST-segment depression
  - "Coving" or "scooped" morphology
  - Concave upward
- T wave changes
  - Decreased amplitude; flattening
  - Inversion
  - Biphasic
- QT interval shortening
- Prominent U waves
- PR segment lengthening (maybe minor)

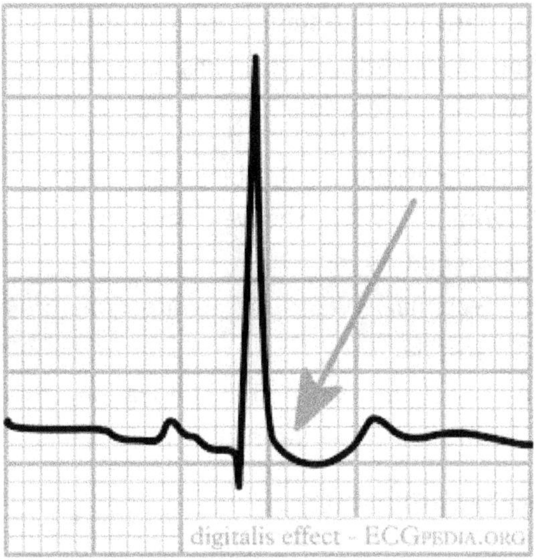

DIGOXIN TOXICITY:

Almost any type of arrhythmia can be observed.

The most common arrhythmia which is observed in digoxin intoxication is premature ventricular systole (PVS) uniquely bidirectional PVS

Digoxin depresses conduction in the atrioventricular node or AV-node and may result in:

- AV blocks
- Sinus bradycardia
- Sinoatrial exit blocks

Atrial tachycardias or ventricular tachycardias are seen.

Ventricular tachycardias may be monomorphic VT as well as bidirectional VT.

There is no particular ECG finding for digoxin intoxication, but observation of any of the following ECG findings strongly suggests digoxin intoxication:

- Atrial tachycardia with a block: atrial rate is more than 100/minute while the ventricular rate is less than 100/minute.
- Bidirectional VPS or bidirectional ventricular tachycardia.
- In a patient with atrial fibrillation, there is an Equalization of R-R intervals.

Managing Digoxin toxicity:

- Digoxin should be withdrawn immediately.
- Verapamil, spironolactone, diltiazem, amiodarone, or carvedilol are the Drugs that may increase serum levels of digoxin, so these should be withdrawn immediately.
- Hypokalemia, if present, should be corrected. Hypokalemia exacerbates arrhythmias in digoxin intoxication.
- Hypokalemia is frequently observed in patients using diuretics as the treatment of heart failure.
- If there is no hemodynamic instability, removal of digoxin and observing the cardiac rhythm is usually enough.
- A temporary cardiac pacemaker may be implanted if there is AV block and syncope.
- Digoxin-specific Fab-fragments act immediately. It is ideal for patients with life-threatening arrhythmias.

- If ventricular arrhythmias are observed, Antiarrhythmic drugs should be used. However, remember that antiarrhythmic medications may cause or worsen AV block while suppressing ventricular arrhythmias.
- In patients with digoxin intoxication, Electrical cardioversion may result in ventricular fibrillation or asystole, so it is relatively contraindicated in these patients.

Calcium channel blockade

Severe calcium channel blocker toxicity is very lethal, as a result of cardiovascular collapse but Good outcomes can be accomplished through aggressive treatment and provision of circulatory support

MECHANISM OF TOXICITY

- Verapamil and diltiazem are highly lethal calcium-channel blockers in case of overdose
- Calcium channel blockers bind with the alpha-1 subunit of L-type calcium channels, preventing the intracellular influx of calcium
- These channels are functionally crucial for cardiac myocytes, vascular smooth muscle cells, and islet beta cells of the pancreas.
- In overdose, receptor selectivity is lost, so even dihydropyridines (e.g., amlodipine) may cause

cardiotoxicity in addition to vasodilation in massive overdoses.

SIGNS AND SYMPTOMS:

Signs and symptoms of calcium channels blockers toxicity:

- Dizziness or lightheadedness
- Weakness
- Syncope
- Chest pain
- Palpitations
- Diaphoresis
- Flushing
- Peripheral edema
- Dyspnea
- Confusion
- Seizure
- Headache
- Nausea and vomiting

Physical examination findings may include the following:

- Slowed heart rate
- Hypotension
- Depressed level of consciousness

Hyperglycaemia, as well as hypoglycemia, may occur. (severity often correlates with the severity of toxicity of calcium channel blockers.)

EKG findings in case of toxicity:

On ECG, toxicity from calcium channel blockers may manifest as following

- Bradycardia
- First-, second-, or third-degree atrioventricular (AV) block
- Any bundle-branch block
- Nonspecific ST-T wave changes

Management:

1-Stabilize airway, breathing, and circulation (ABCs)

2-Correction of acid-base disturbances and electrolyte abnormalities

3-recommended duration of clinical observation for asymptomatic patients with significant exposure to CCBs is as follows:

- Immediate-release products: 6 hours
- Standard-release products: 6-12 hours
- Extended-release or once-a-day preparations: 24-36 hours

4-Activated charcoal has been demonstrated to significantly absorb immediate-release medications within 1 hour of ingestion and extended-release medications as long as four hours after ingestion

The 5-Consult regional poison control center in all cases to assist in the management

6-Specific agents used in treatment include the following:

- Intravenous Normal saline or Ringer lactate for volume expansion.
- Intravenous Calcium
- Intravenous Glucagon
- Vasopressors (e.g., dopamine, epinephrine, norepinephrine)
- High-dose insulin/euglycemia (HIE) therapy
- Lipid emulsion therapy
- Cardiac pacing may be required.

Beta-adrenergic receptor blockade

Beta-blockers: Atenolol, metoprolol, propranolol, sotalol.

Effects on the ECG

- Sinus bradycardia.
- Junctional bradycardia.
- AV blocks (1st degree, 2nd degree, and 3rd degree).
- Ventricular bradycardia.
- Idioventricular rhythm
- Asystole

  A prolonged PR interval is an early sign of beta-blocker

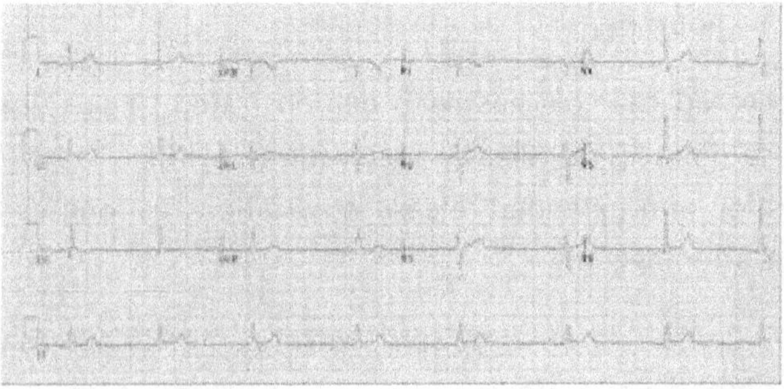

Propanolol:

- Propranolol behaves more like a tricyclic antidepressant in overdose than a beta-blocker, due to its blockade of myocardial and CNS fast sodium channels.
- Propranolol toxicity is associated with QRS widening and a positive R' wave in aVR (signs of sodium channel blockade), which portend the onset of coma, seizures, hypotension, and ventricular arrhythmias.

Sotalol

Sotalol blocks myocardial potassium channels, causing QT prolongation and Torsades de Pointes in overdose.

CHAPTER 17:
EKG CHANGES IN CONGENITAL HEART DISEASES:
ACYANOTIC HEART DISEASES:

acyanotic congenital heart defects include:

- Ventricular septal defect (VSD).
- Atrial septal defect (ASD).
- Atrioventricular septal defect.
- Patent ductus arteriosus (PDA).
- Pulmonary valve stenosis.
- Aortic valve stenosis.
- Coarctation of the aorta.
- Pulmonary regurgitation
- Aortic regurgitation
- Mitral valve prolapse
- Mitral valve regurgitation
- Mitral valve stenosis

Ventral septal defects

It is a congenital birth defect in which interventricular septum is deficient. It may occur in adults after myocardial infarction. Its frequency is 15% to 20% of all cardiac defects which makes VSD is the most common congenital heart defect

A VSD may occur as the primary anomaly with or without additional significant associated cardiac abnormalities.

The ventricular septal defect could be in any part of the ventricular septum (small membranous portion and a large muscular portion. The inlet defect is located beneath the tricuspid valve while the outlet defect is located at the sub-pulmonary part of the ventricular septum.

The defects vary in size, ranging from minute defects without hemodynamic significance to significant defects with accompanying CHF and pulmonary hypertension.

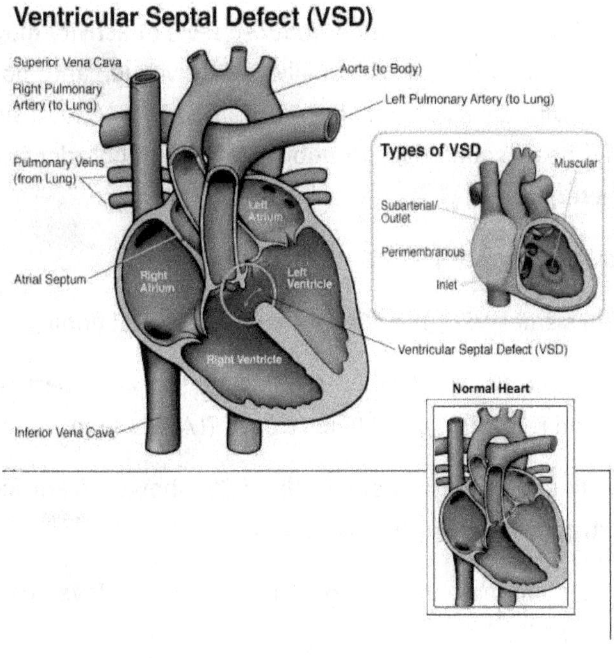

CLINICAL MANIFESTATIONS

1. With a small VSD, the patient is usually healthy and asymptomatic with normal growth and development. The characteristic harsh, holosystolic murmur is loudest at the lower left sternal border (LSB), and it is well localized.

2. With a moderate to large VSD, poor growth, delayed development, reduced exercise tolerance, repeated pulmonary infections, and CHF is relatively common during infancy. A holosystolic harsh murmur is most prominent at the lower LSB. The intensity of the pulmonary component is typically normal or slightly increased.

3. With long-standing pulmonary hypertension, the patient presents with cyanosis, and a reduced level of activity may be present. The murmur is usually short, vague, and poorly located with an accompanying diastolic rumble. A loud single second heart sound over the upper left sternal border is also characteristic.

Electrocardiography

1. With a small VSD, the ECG has no pathological finding.

2. With a moderate VSD, mostly left ventricular hypertrophy (LVH) and rarely left atrial hypertrophy (LAH) is seen.

3. With a significant defect, the ECG shows biventricular hypertrophy (BVH) with or without LAH.

4. If the pulmonary vascular obstructive disease develops, the ECG shows RVH only

5. RBBB (right bundle branch block) may occur in patients with VSD after repair by right ventriculotomy. It usually occurs due to the disruption of the Purkinje fibers or direct injury to the right bundle itself.

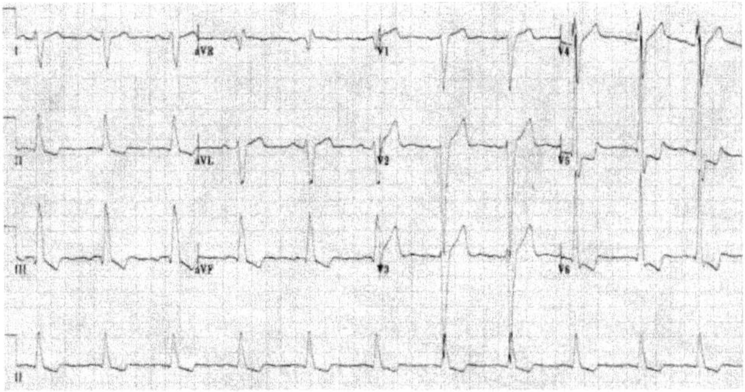

Above EKG is showing biventricular hypertrophy.

Management:

- Treatment of CHF, if it develops, needs treatment with digoxin and diuretics
- good dental hygiene and antibiotic prophylaxis for infective endocarditis is essential
- the VSD should be operated within the first six months of life if Small infants, who have large VSDs and develop CHF along with growth retardation, which is not improving by medical therapy
- Infants with evidence of pulmonary hypertension but no CHF or growth failure should have a cardiac catheterization at 6 to 12 months of age, and Surgery should be followed soon after that.

Atrial septal defect

Atrial septal defect (ASD) is a congenital heart defect in which there is communication between the atria (upper chambers) of the heart through a defect in the inter-atrial septum.

Ostium secundum ASD is the most frequent type of ASD (5-10%), which involves the fossa ovalis in the mid-septal region.

Ostium primum type of ASD is a rare defect is near tricuspid valves. In an atrioventricular septal defect, the tricuspid valves are also deformed.

Occasionally a defect that is seen high in the atrial septum near the entry of superior venacava (SVC) is known as Sinus venosus type. It might also present near to inferior vena cava.

Coronary sinus type is another type of ASD, involving the roof of the coronary sinus

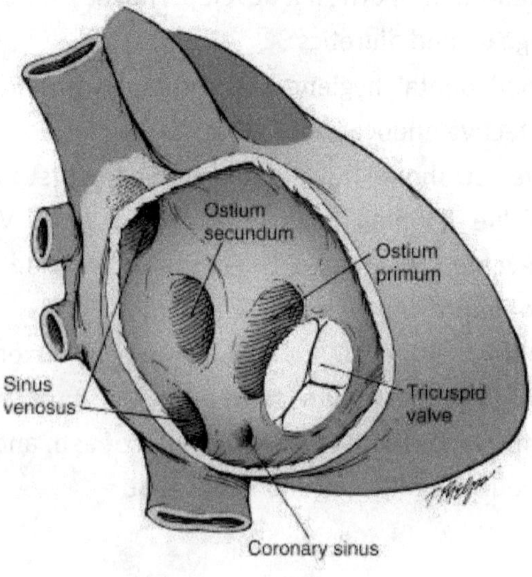

Clinical presentation:

- a widely split and fixed S2(second heart sound) and ejection systolic murmur of grade 2 to 3/6 are characteristic findings of ASD in older infants and children.
- these findings might not be present unless the shunt is reasonably large
- most of the time, the patient is asymptomatic.

Electrocardiography

- +90 to +180 degrees Right axis deviation.
- Right ventricular hypertrophy (RVH) is usually mild.
- Right bundle branch block (RBBB) and an rsR' pattern in V1.
- In about 50% of the patients with sinus venosus ASD, the P axis is less than 30 degrees.

ECG

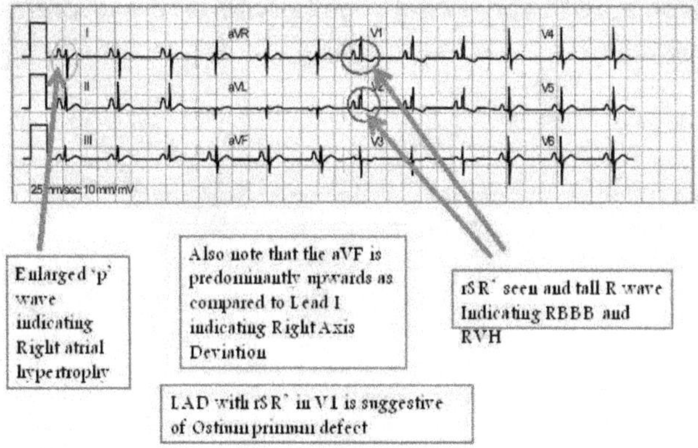

Management:

- In infants with CHF, manage accordingly
- Several closure devices can be delivered via cardiac catheters. These are safe and efficient for ASD closure. These devices apply only to secundum ASD
- surgery is performed during infancy only If CHF does not respond to medical treatment or if device closure is considered inappropriate.

Patent Ductus Arteriosus

There is persistent patency of a normal fetal structure between the left pulmonary artery and the descending aorta. It is located 5 to 10 mm, distal to the base of the left subclavian artery.

The ductus is usually cone-shaped with a small orifice to the PA, which is restrictive to blood flow. The ductus may be straight or tortuous, short or long

male/female ratio is of 1:3 (It is more common in females than in males). PDA is a common problem in patients with Down Syndrome, with congenital rubella syndrome and premature infants.

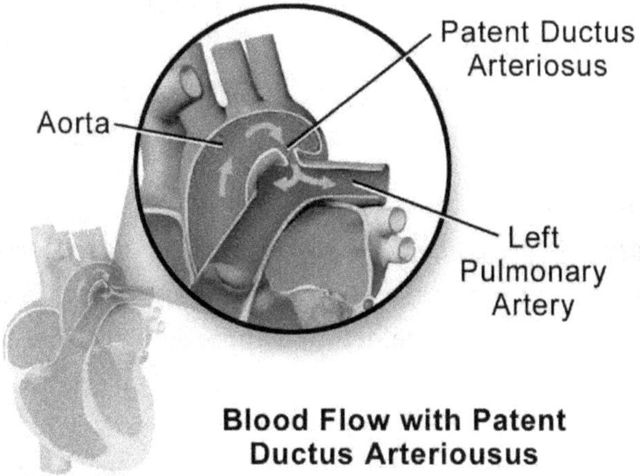

Blood Flow with Patent Ductus Arteriousus

Clinical presentation:

Patients are usually asymptomatic with the small-shunt ductus arteriosus. But lower respiratory tract infection, atelectasis, exertional dyspnea, and CHF are common in large shunt PDA.

On clinical examination, there will be bounding peripheral pulses with the hyperdynamic pericardium. The P2 is usually of normal intensity, but it may become loud if pulmonary hypertension is present. A continuous murmur or machinery murmur, of grade 1 to 4/6, is best audible at the left infraclavicular area or left upper sternal border.

ECG FINDINGS:

- The ECG results are usually the same as VSD.
- A normal ECG or LVH is found with small to moderate size PDA.
- BVH is seen with large PDA.

- If the pulmonary vascular obstructive disease develops, RVH is present.
- In preterm infants, the ECG is not diagnostic. It is usually normal but occasionally shows LVH.

Atrioventricular septal defect

It is also known as the atrioventricular canal (AVC) defects and endocardial cushion defect (ECD). They account for 4% to 5% of all congenital heart defects and approximately 0.5% of live births. AVSDs are found to have a strong association with Trisomy 21 (DOWN SYNDROME) and complete asplenia. Non-syndromic AV canal defects are associated with maternal diabetes and obesity.

In this defect, there is an inadequate fusion of the endocardial cushions with the muscular portion of the ventricular septum and middle part of the atrial septum.

There are two common types of AVSDs, complete and partial.

In Partial AVSD (primum ASD), the lower part of the atrial septum is defective. It is also associated with a split anterior mitral leaflet, causing mitral insufficiency. The ventricular septum is usually intact.

Complete AVSD has a defect that stretches from the lower part of the atrial septum to the upper part (inlet) of the interventricular septum. Due to this deficiency, both the mitral valve and tricuspid valve are attached to form a common AV valve, that overhangs the interventricular septum.

CLINICAL MANIFESTATIONS

Patients will present with complaints of Failure to thrive, repeated respiratory infections, and signs of congestive heart failure.

A holosystolic murmur, of grade 3 to 4/6, is usually best heard at the lower left sternal border. The systolic murmur may transmit to the back on the left side.

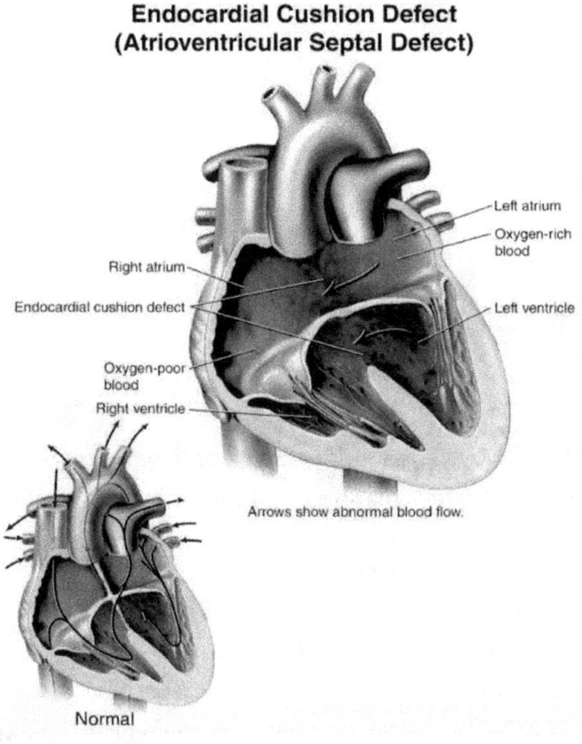

Electrocardiography

1. the QRS axis between -40 and -150 degrees, also known as the "Superior" QRS axis, is characteristic of this defect. Left

superior axis deviation is due to anatomical displacement of AV-node in the inferior and posterior direction.

2. Most of the patients have a long PR interval (first-degree AV block), probably due to abnormal AV node conduction.

3. In all cases, RVH or RBBB is present.

4. LVH is also a common finding among many patients(due to increased pressure).

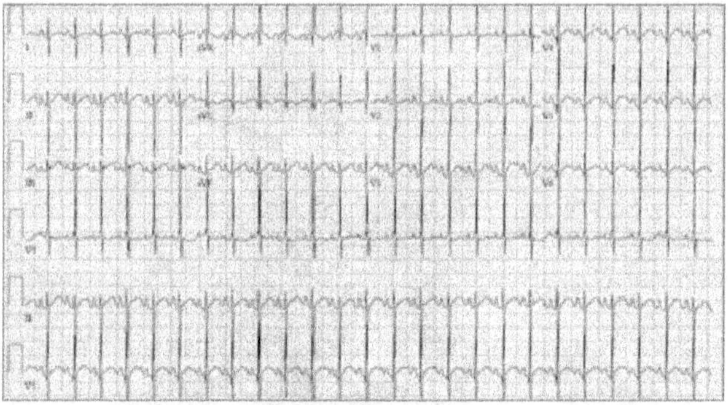

In AVSD, there is Left superior QRS axis deviation (negative in aVF) and right ventricular hypertrophy.

Pulmonary Stenosis (PS)

- Pulmonary stenosis can be valvular, infundibular or subvalvular, and supravalvular.
- The valvular PS is the commonest form.
- In the Tetralogy of Fallot, Infundibular PS has usually associated with VSD.
- In Williams syndrome and congenital rubella, there is pulmonary stenosis of supravalvular type.

- Supravalvular PS may occur as a complication of a previous arterial switch surgery.
- Peripheral pulmonary artery stenosis may occur due to congenital rubella or associated Alagille or Noonan syndromes.

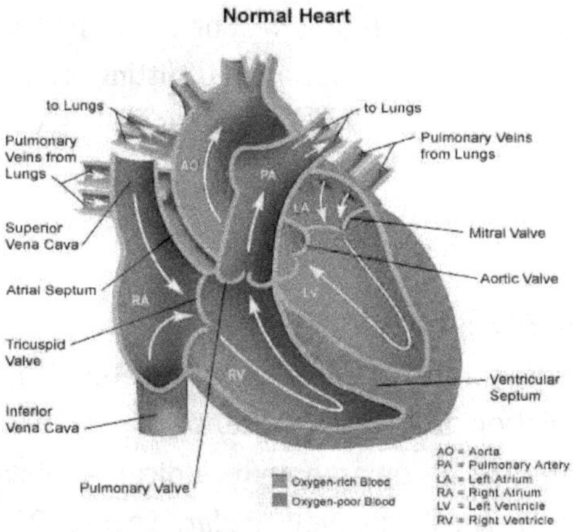

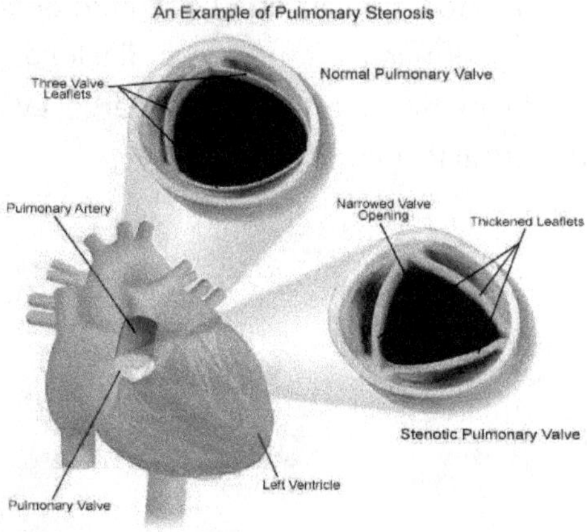

Clinical presentations:

Patients with mild or moderate pulmonary stenosis are usually asymptomatic.

Severe PS may present with symptoms of decreased cardiac output such as exertional dyspnea and, subsequently, symptoms of congestive cardiac failure.

An ejection systolic murmur is best heard at the ULSB radiating to the back. Wide (and variable) splitting of second heart sound is commonly present. In the case of valvular stenosis, ejection click can also be heard.

Electrocardiography:

- The EKG is normal in mild PS.
- In moderate or severe cases, RVH and right axis deviation are usually present.
- Right atrial enlargement indicates elevated filling pressure of right ventricular. Severe PS may cause deep inverted T wave and ST-segment depression(RV strain pattern) in the right precordial leads.
- Because of hypoplastic RV and large LV, newborns with critical PS may show LVH.

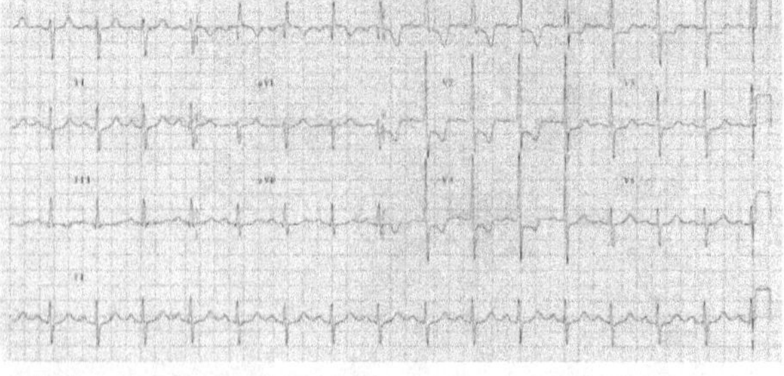

RVH and right ventricular strain pattern in EKG

Mitral stenosis

It is a valvular heart disease characterized by the narrowing of the orifice of the mitral valve of the heart

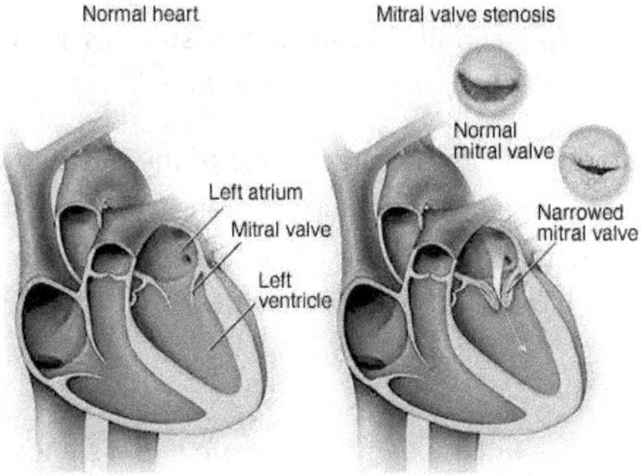

Rheumatic fever is the most frequent reason for mitral stenosis. There is an association between atrial septal defect with rheumatic mitral stenosis known as Lutembacher syndrome. Other, less common etiologies for mitral stenosis include malignant carcinoid disease, systemic lupus erythematosus, rheumatoid arthritis.

Signs and symptoms of mitral stenosis are as following:

- Heart failure symptoms, such as exertional dyspnea, orthopnea and paroxysmal nocturnal dyspnea (PND)
- Palpitations
- Chest pain
- Hemoptysis
- Thromboembolism in later stages

- Ascites and edema and hepatomegaly (if right-side heart failure develops)
- Fatigue and weakness increase with exercise and pregnancy

The presence of mitral facies (pinkish-purple patches on the cheeks) indicates chronic severe mitral stenosis leading to reduced cardiac output and vasoconstriction.

The auscultatory findings characteristic of mitral stenosis is a loud first heart sound, an opening snap, and a diastolic rumble best heard at the apex in the left lateral position. Murmur decreases with rest and Valsalva maneuver.

ECG findings:

On ECG, patients with moderate-to-severe mitral stenosis may show the following :

- P-wave, of duration >0.12 seconds in the lead II, indicating Left atrial enlargement.
- P wave axis is of +45 to -30 degree.
- The most commonly found arrhythmias is Atrial fibrillation
- A mean QRS axis indicates the presence of right ventricular hypertrophy in the frontal plane of >80 degrees, and an R-to-S ratio of >1 in lead V1.
- The mean QRS axis moves toward the right in the frontal plane, with the increasing severity of pulmonary hypertension.

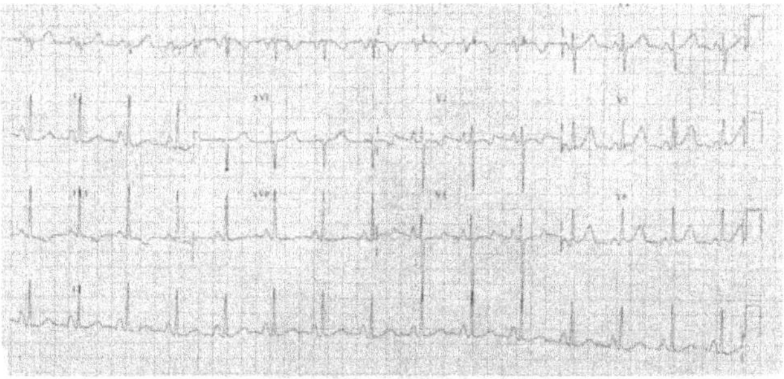

Aortic Stenosis (AS)

- Aortic stenosis, the aortic valve becomes narrow.
- In this condition, there is a restriction of the blood flow from the left ventricle to the aorta. It may also affect the pressure in the left atrium.
- Aortic stenosis may be valvular, supravalvular or sub-valvular
- In Williams syndrome and after arterial switch procedure for D-TGA, supravalvularAS can be found.
- There is sub-valvular obstruction with a discrete fibrous ring or membrane, causing severe blood flow limitation.
- The bicuspid aortic valve is a common cause of AS in patients with Turner Syndrome.
- It is more common in males.

Normal Heart

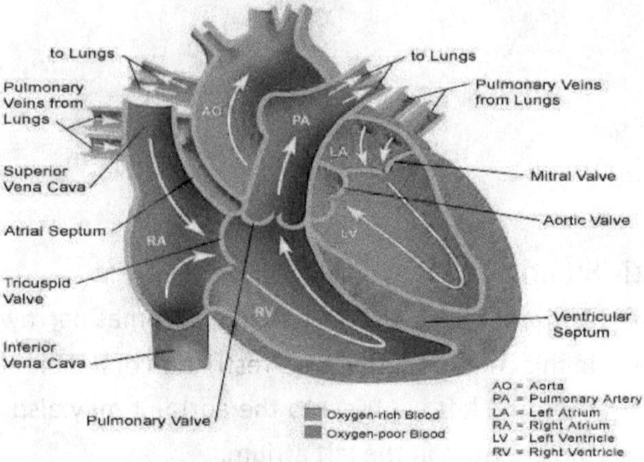

An Example of Aortic Stenosis

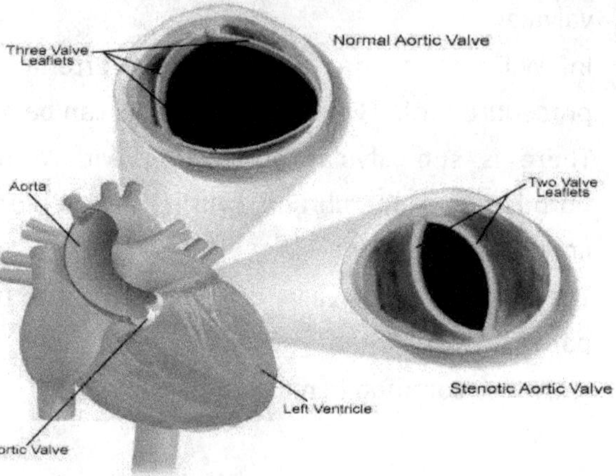

Clinical presentations:

- mild or moderate aortic stenosis(AS) is usually asymptomatic.
- Severe AS may be accompanied by exertional dyspnea, and chest pain with decreased exercise tolerance, or episodes of syncope.
- Infants with critical AS may present with congestive cardiac failure early in life.
- In severe AS, The pulse pressure may be narrow.
- In supra-valvular AS, there is higher BP in the right arm than the left, due to preferential streaming (Coanda effect) to the subclavian artery of the right side.
- The presence of a regular or accentuated A2 speaks against the existence of severe aortic stenosis. The usual finding is diminished or absent A2.
- Paradoxical splitting of the S2: Resulting from late closure of the aortic valve with delayed A2
- the presence of secondary pulmonary hypertension, there is Accentuated of the pulmonary component of the second heart sound.
- In children and young adults, Ejection click is a common finding.
- Forceful contraction of atria into a hypertrophied left ventricle results in prominent fourth heart sound.
- An ejection systolic murmur is best heard at the upper left and right sternal border and radiates to the carotid arteries.

Electrocardiography:

- EKG is usually normal in mild AS
- LVH indicates moderate or severe AS
- inverted T waves (strain pattern)may be seen in left precordial leads.
- Atrial fibrillation can be seen at late stages.
- Ambulatory ECG monitoring frequently shows complex ventricular arrhythmias, particularly in cases with myocardial dysfunction.

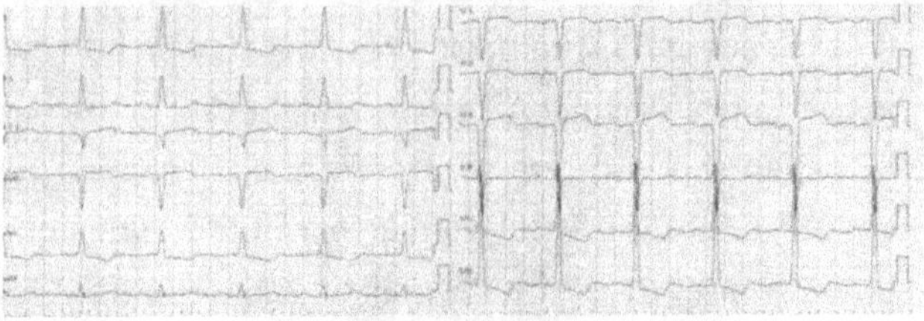

Normal Heart

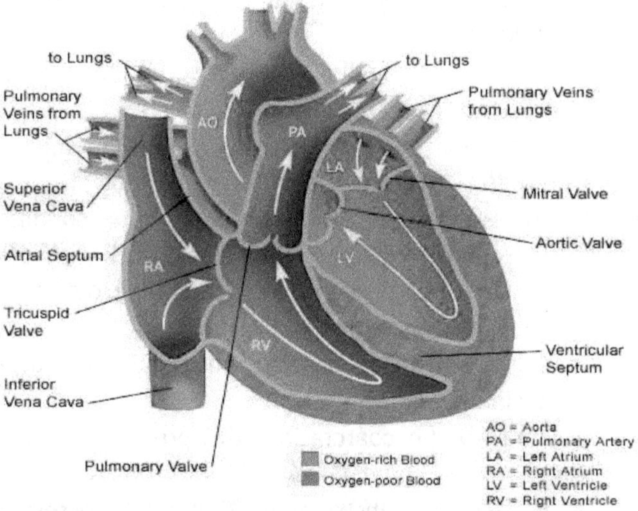

Coarctation of the Aorta

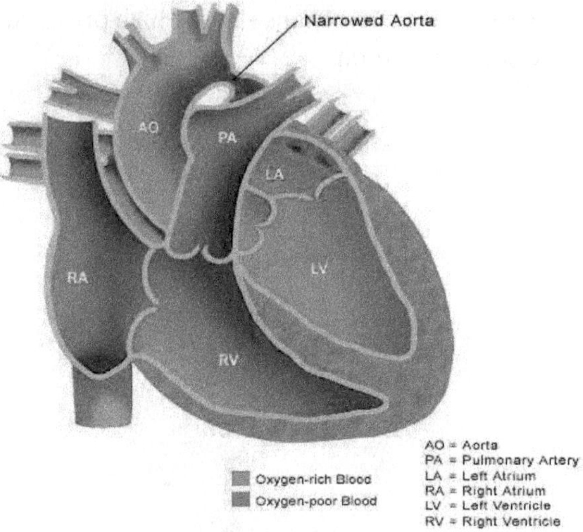

Coarctation of the Aorta

- occurrences of COA is 8% to 10% of all the congenital heart defect.
- Males are more affected by this condition than females (male/female ratio of 2:1).
- Coarctation of the aorta can be both congenital and acquired(in Takayasu arteritis)
- It may also be associated with some other conditions like Turner or Williams syndromes, and with other congenital heart diseases such as double outlet right ventricle, bicuspid aortic valve, VSD.
- Coarctation of the aorta causes mechanical obstacle in blood circulation.
- Proximal to the coarctation, the pressure is usually high.
- To bypass the obstruction, Collateral vessels are formed, and the most common collaterals are between the internal mammary and the intercostal arteries.
- LVH develops in response to the high pressure proximal to the coarctation.

<u>Coarctation of aorta</u>

Types

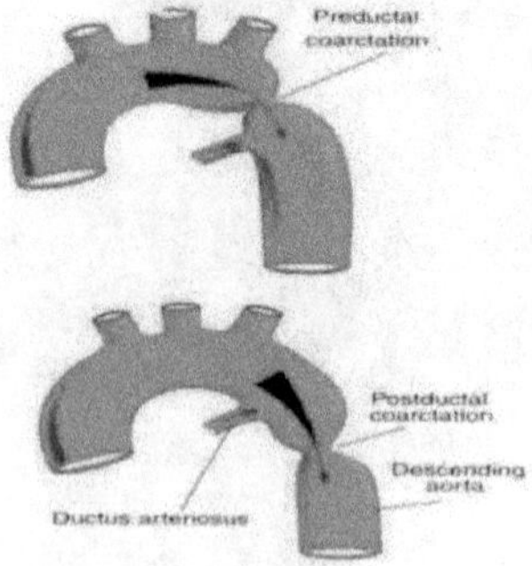

Clinical Presentation

- Most patients with coarctation are asymptomatic.
- Some patients may present with symptoms of upper extremity hypertension like headaches, blurred vision, or frequent nosebleeds.
- Typical signs of reduced blood flow to the lower extremities are exercise-induced claudication, Oliguria or anuria, general circulatory shock, and severe acidemia.
- In infancy, as the ductus arteriosus closes, severe coarctation may present with CHF.
- Differential cyanosis may be present; for instance, only the lower half of the body is cyanotic because of a right-to-left ductal shunt.

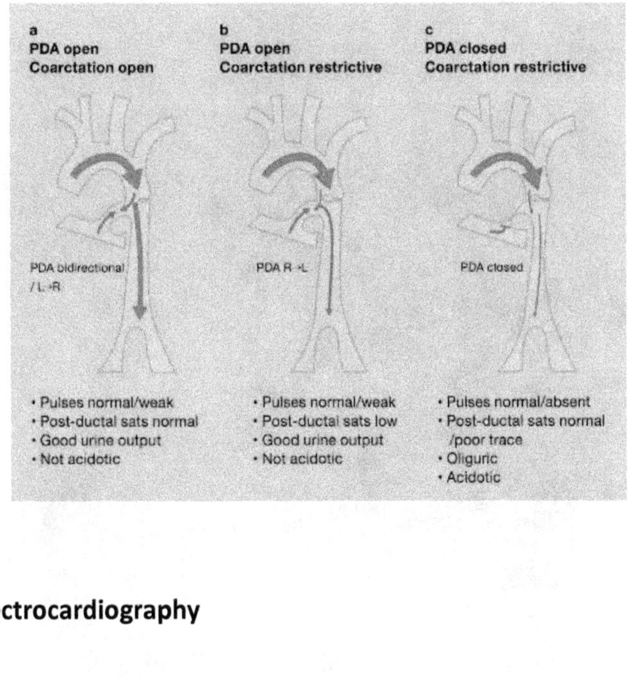

Electrocardiography

- A standard or rightward QRS axis and RVH or right bundle branch block (RBBB) are present in most infants with COA.
- LVH is seen in older children (2nd or 3rd year of life).
- The ECG appears normal in 20% of patients.

Pulmonary regurgitation

Pulmonary insufficiency (or incompetence, or regurgitation) is a condition in which the pulmonary valve is incompetent and allows the backflow of blood from the pulmonary artery to the right ventricle of the heart during diastole. Pulmonary valvular insufficiency is most often due to other cardiovascular diseases or may be secondary to severe pulmonary hypertension.

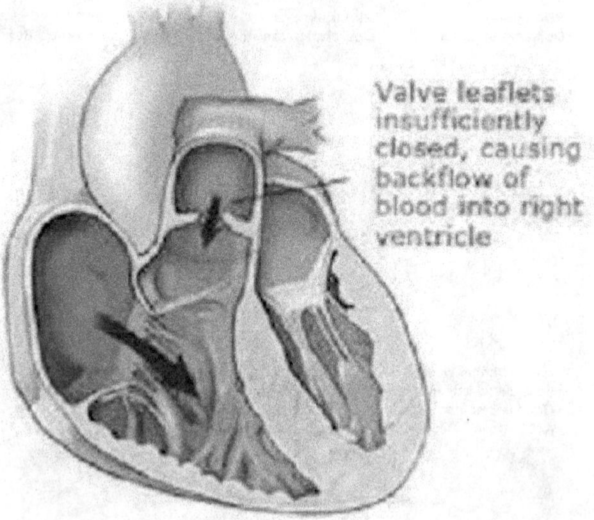

Among the causes of pulmonary insufficiency are:

- Infective endocarditis
- Rheumatic heart disease
- Connective tissue disease
- Carcinoid syndrome
- Congestive abnormalities
- Prosthetic heart valve

The incompetence of the valve occurs after surgery, like after pulmonary valvotomy in patients with valvular pulmonic stenosis or patients with tetralogy of Fallot after valvotomy with infundibular resection.

Isolated congenital insufficiency of the pulmonary valve is a rare finding. These patients are usually asymptomatic.

Jugular venous pressure (JVP) is usually increased. Often, an increased A wave is present. The prominent physical sign is a low-pitched diastolic murmur at the left upper and mid-left sternal border.

The electrocardiogram (ECG) is normal or shows the following changes

- **qR pattern or Tall R wave in V1.**
- **In V1, R-wave is bigger than S wave**
- **In the right precordial leads (V1, V2), an rSR' pattern.**
- **R wave progression reversal in the precordial leads**
- **In the anterior precordial leads, there are Inverted T wave**
- **Right axis deviation**

- **minimal RV hypertrophy**
- **Right atrial enlargement**

Mitral insufficiency

It is a form of valvular heart disease in which the mitral valve does not close appropriately when the heart pumps out blood. It is the abnormal leaking of blood backward from the left ventricle, through the mitral valve, into the left atrium. Congenital mitral insufficiency is rarely a solitary lesion. It is also known as Mitral regurgitation (MR), mitral insufficiency, and mitral incompetence.

It is most frequently encountered in combination with

- an atrioventricular septal defect.
- dilated cardiomyopathy
- with coarctation of the aorta
- VSD
- corrected transposition of the great vessels
- from the pulmonary artery, there is the anomalous origin of the left coronary artery.
- Marfan syndrome.

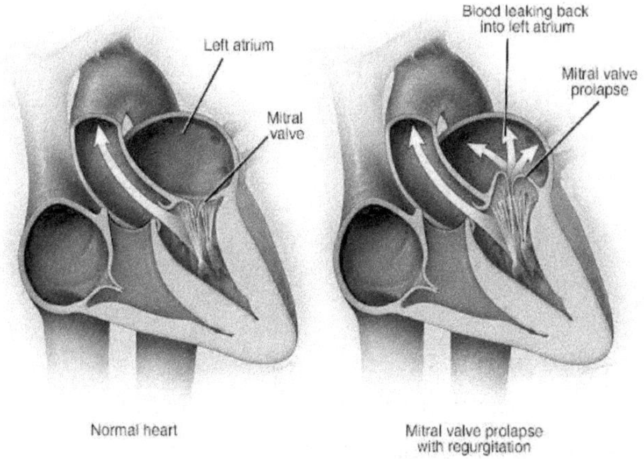

In the absence of other congenital heart diseases, endocarditis or rheumatic fever should be suspected in a patient with isolated severe mitral insufficiency

Signs and symptoms are of acute decompensated congestive heart failure (i.e., shortness of breath, pulmonary edema, orthopnea, and paroxysmal nocturnal dyspnea), and cardiogenic shock (i.e., shortness of breath at rest).

In acute cases, a systolic murmur is best heard at the base, radiates to the neck, spine, or top of the head while in chronic cases, it is best heard at the apex of the heart and radiates towards the axilla.

The ECG typically demonstrates bifid P waves consistent with left atrial enlargement, signs of LV hypertrophy, and sometimes signs of RV hypertrophy in chronic cases. In acute cases, ECG is usually normal.

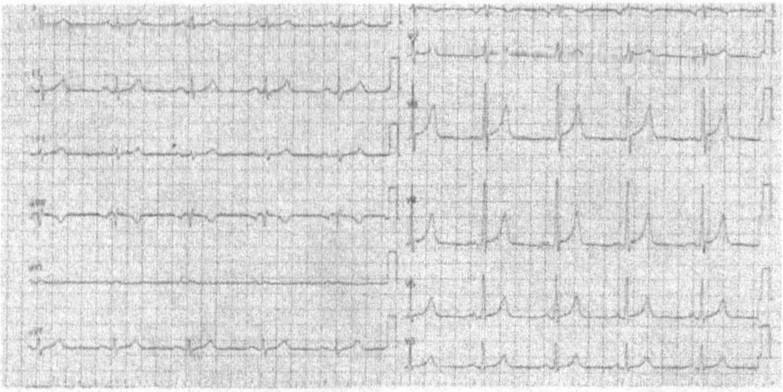

Mitral valve prolapse

Mitral valve prolapse (MVP) is valvular heart disease. MVP is characterized by the displacement of an abnormally thickened mitral valve leaflet in the left atrium during systole. Mitral valve prolapse is frequently accompanying with mild mitral regurgitation

The abnormality is primarily congenital but may not be recognized until adolescence or adulthood.

Mitral valve prolapse is usually sporadic, is more common in girls, and maybe inherited as an autosomal dominant trait.

It is common in patients with Marfan syndrome, straight back syndrome, pectus excavatum, scoliosis, Ehlers-Danlos syndrome, osteogenesis imperfecta, and pseudoxanthoma elasticum. The dominant abnormal signs are auscultatory

Upon auscultation mitral valve prolapse produces a mid-systolic click, followed by a late systolic murmur heard best at the apex, accentuated by standing and Valsalva maneuver

The ECG is usually normal, but in leads II, III, aVF, and V6, it may show biphasic T waves. The T-wave abnormalities may vary in the same patient at different times.

Tricuspid regurgitation

tricuspid regurgitation (TR) is a valvular heart disease in which the tricuspid valve of the heart does not close entirely when the right ventricle contracts during systole. It is also known as Tricuspid insufficiency (TI).

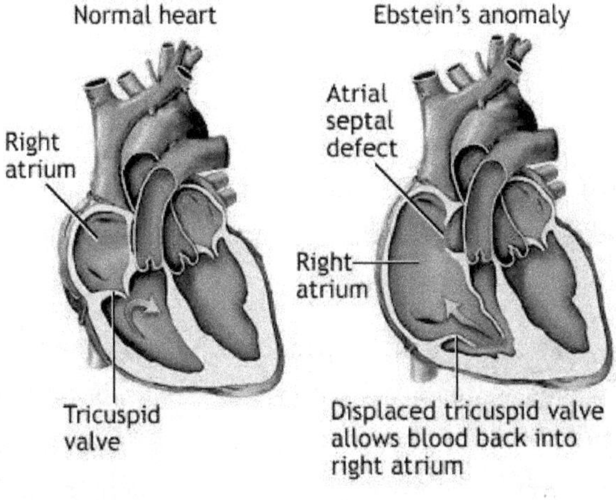

- TR allows the blood to flow backward from the right ventricle to the right atrium, which increases the volume and pressure of the blood both in the right atrium and the right ventricle.
- Isolated tricuspid regurgitation is most often associated with Ebstein anomaly of the tricuspid valve
- Tricuspid regurgitation often accompanies RV dysfunction.

- Tricuspid regurgitation is also encountered in newborns with perinatal asphyxia.
- tricuspid regurgitation is seen in up to 30% of children after heart transplantation

Common presenting complaints of patients with RV dysfunction are:

- Dyspnea on exertion
- Orthopnea
- Paroxysmal nocturnal dyspnea
- Ascites
- Peripheral edema

The high pitched pansystolic murmur is associated with tricuspid regurgitation and is loudest in the fourth intercostal space in the parasternal region.

ECG findings are usually nonspecific. Typical abnormalities are Q waves in lead V1, incomplete right bundle-branch block, and atrial fibrillation.

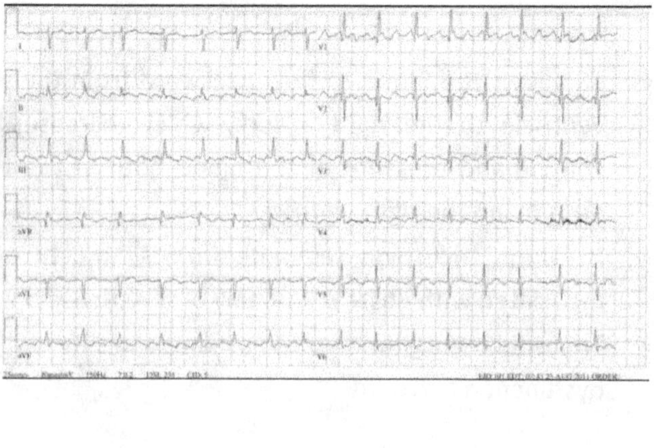

Aortic regurgitation

It is the leaking of the aortic valve of the heart that causes blood to backflow during ventricular diastole.i.e from the aorta into the left ventricle. Aortic regurgitation (AR) is also acknowledged as Aortic insufficiency (AI).

It is more often congenital than acquired in origin

Congenital causes of AR include the following:

- Congenital bicuspid aortic valve
- Following balloon dilatation of the aortic valve
- Associated with ventricular septal defect (either subpulmonary or membranous)
- Secondary to subaortic stenosis
- In association with dilated aortic root (Marfan syndrome or Ehlers-Danlos syndrome)

Rarely, rheumatic heart disease is a cause of AR. AR of rheumatic origin is almost always associated with mitral valve disease as well.

Failure of the aortic valve to close tightly causes back flow of blood into the left ventricle

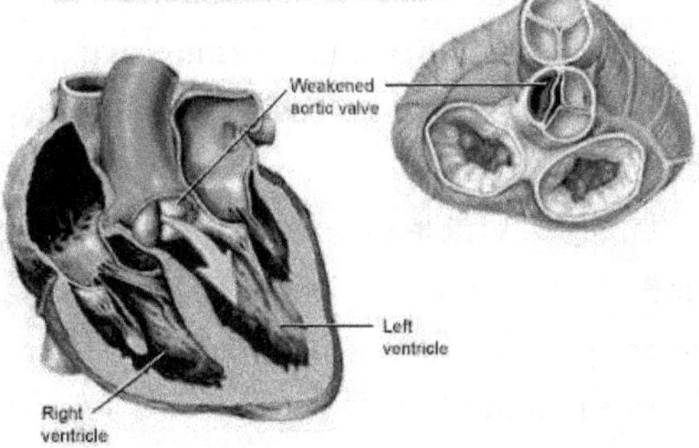

Clinical Manifestations

Symptoms of aortic insufficiency are the same as those of heart failure and include the following:

- Dyspnea on exertion
- Orthopnea
- Paroxysmal nocturnal dyspnea
- Palpitations
- Angina pectoris
- Cyanosis (in acute cases)

Associated physical examination findings include the following:

- Visible systolic pulsations of the retinal arterioles are known as Becker sign.
- Bobbing motion of the patient's head with every heartbeat is known as de Musset sign.
- Popliteal cuff systolic blood pressure is of 40 mm Hg or higher than brachial cuff systolic blood pressure is known as Hill sign.
- Systolic murmur over the femoral artery, auscultated with the stethoscope, after proximal compression of the artery and diastolic murmur over the femoral artery with distal compression of the artery is known as Duroziez sign.
- Müller sign - Visible systolic pulsations of the uvula
- Sudden distension and instant collapse on palpation of the peripheral arterial pulse is known as Corrigan pulse ("water-hammer" pulse).

- Visible pulsations at the fingernail bed, with light compression of the fingernail, is known as Quincke sign.
- Booming systolic and diastolic sounds heard over the femoral artery with a stethoscope is known as a Traube sign or"pistol-shot" pulse.

The murmur of AR occurs in diastole, usually as a high-pitched sound that is loudest at the left sternal border.

Electrocardiography:

- The ECG is normal in mild cases.
- In severe cases, LVH is usually present.
- LAH may be present in long-standing cases.
- In leads I, aVL, and V3-V6, Prominent Q waves and in Lead V1 comparatively small r waves (LV volume overload pattern)
- LV conduction defects - Typically appear late in the disease process.

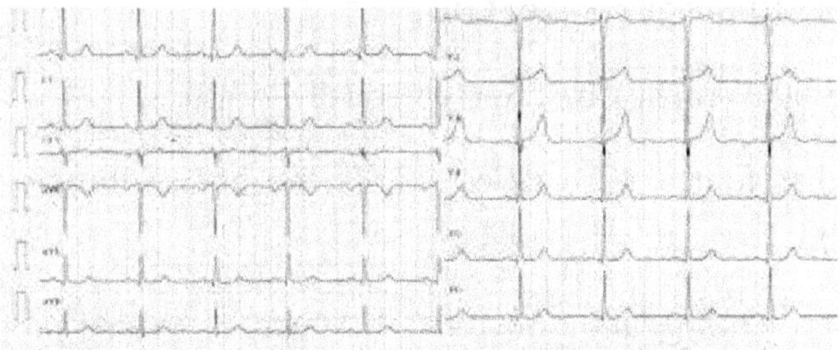

Cyanotic Cardiac Lesions:

Cyanosis is the purplish or bluish discoloration of the skin or mucous membranes due to low oxygen saturation in the tissues situated below the skin.

List of Cyanotic congenital heart defects are as follows,

- Tetralogy of Fallot
- Tricuspid atresia
- Total anomalous pulmonary venous return
- Truncus arteriosus
- Transposition of great arteries
- Hypoplastic left heart syndrome
- Ebstein anomaly

Tetralogy of Fallot (TOF)

Among cyanotic heart diseases, the Tetralogy of Fallot is one of the most common ones.

It includes more than 50% of all cases of with cyanotic CHD and overall 10% of all cases of CHD

Males and females are affected equally.

TOF has four abnormalities (hence the phrase 'tetralogy is used):

- Ventricular septal defect (mal-alignment, nonrestrictive, perimembranous)
- Overriding aorta

- infundibular stenosis or overgrowth of the heart muscle wall leading to Right ventricular outflow tract obstruction (RVOTO).
- Right ventricular hypertrophy (RVH)

other anatomical anomalies which may present with Tetralogy of Fallot are following

- in 40% of cases, there is stenosis of the left pulmonary artery
- in 60% of cases, there is a bicuspid pulmonary valve with Tetralogy of Fallot.
- right-sided aortic arch, in 25%
- coronary artery anomalies, in 10%
- pentalogy of Fallot (Tetralogy of Fallot with a patent foramen ovale or atrial septal defect)
- an atrioventricular septal defect
- partial or total anomalous pulmonary venous return
- pseudotruncus arteriosus (Tetralogy of Fallot with pulmonary atresia) is a severe variant

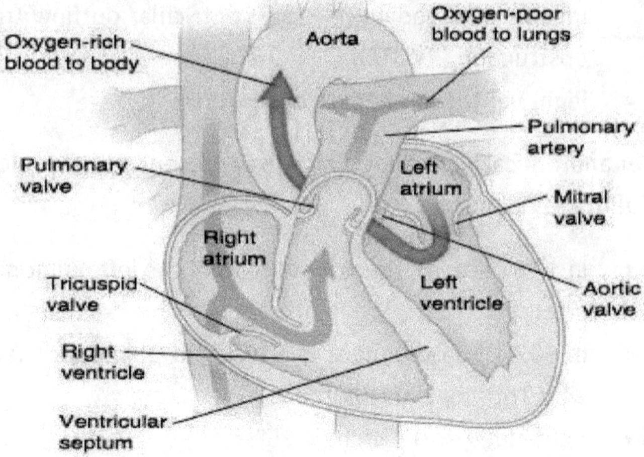

In a normal heart, oxygen-poor blood is pumped to the lungs from the right ventricle. Oxygen-rich blood is pumped to the body from the left ventricle.

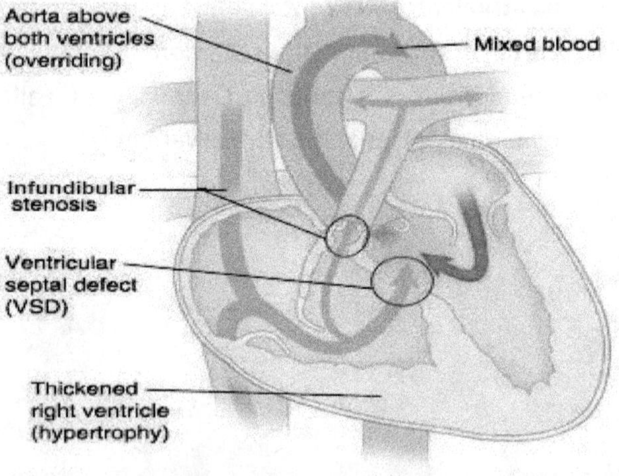

With TOF, there is reduced blood flow from the heart to the lungs.

Clinical presentations:

- Most patients are symptomatic with cyanosis since birth or shortly after that.
- Even in mildly cyanotic infants, dyspnea on exertion, squatting, or hypoxic spells develop later on.
- Infants and children develop hypoxic spells known as **"tet spells"** if the tetralogy of Fallot is not repaired on time. **Tet spells** are characterized by shortness of breath (dyspnea), cyanosis, agitation, and loss of consciousness even fits. Any event such as anxiety, pain, dehydration, or fever can initiate it.
- In older infants and children, varying degrees of cyanosis, tachypnea, and clubbing are present.
- There is a right ventricular heave at the left parasternal border (due to the right ventricular hypertrophy, ejection systolic murmur (due to RVOTO), and single Second heart sound (due to pulmonary hypertension).

The cause is typically not known, but risk factors include,

- Alcoholic mother
- Diabetic mother
- a mother is over the age of 40
- rubella infection during pregnancy
- It may also be associated with Down-syndrome.

Electrocardiography

1. In cyanotic TOF, Right axis deviation (RAD) of +120 to +150 degrees is present

2. The QRS axis is normal in acyanotic patients.

3. Despite RVH, strain pattern is not usual because RV pressure is not supra systemic.

4. BVH may be seen in acyanotic patients.

5. RAH is occasionally present.

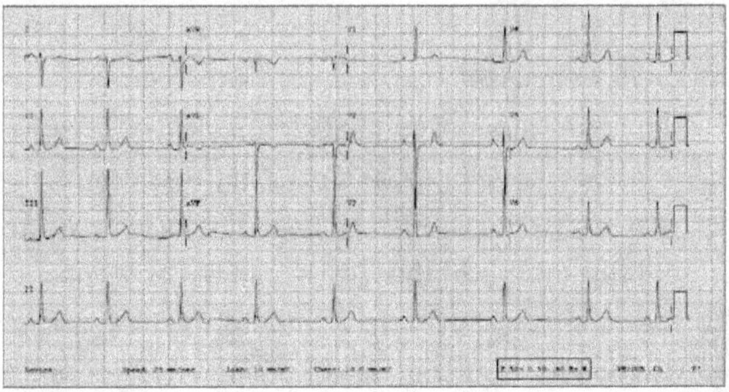

Electrocardiogram (ECG) reveals normal sinus rhythm, right axis deviation, and right ventricular hypertrophy with monophasic R wave in V1 and transition to rS in V2.

Treatment:

Surgical correction of the defect is always essential. Corrective repair of the tetralogy of Fallot involves

- To normal blood flow from the left ventricle to the aorta, closure of the ventricular septal defect is done with a synthetic Dacron patch.

- The narrowing of the pulmonary valve and right ventricular outflow tract is enlarged by cutting away the obstructive muscle tissue in the right ventricle and by expanding the outflow pathway with a patch.

Following ECG is done in a patient who had undergone corrective surgery of TOF.ECG is demonstrating normal sinus rhythm with a complete right bundle branch block and a QRS duration of 178 ms.

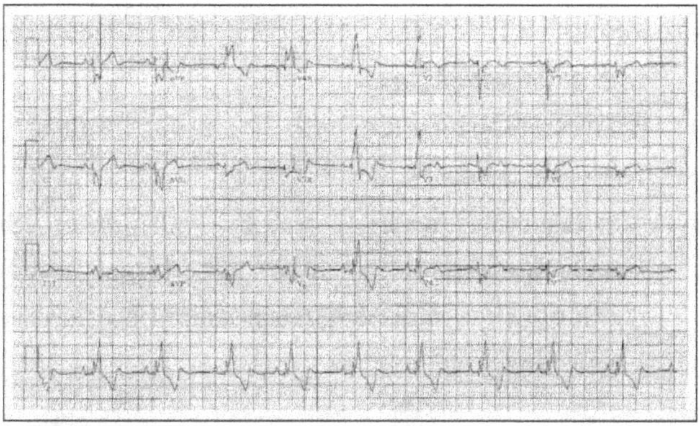

Tricuspid Atresia (TA)

- TA is a rare form of CHD.
- Its frequency is 1% of all CHD.
- The tricuspid valve is absent
- the RV is hypoplastic, with an absence of the inflow portion of the RV.
- ASD, VSD, or PDA are essential for survival in patients with tricuspid atresia
- The pulmonary valve would also be atretic in case of the intact ventricular septum.

- Therc will be a variable degree of pulmonary valve hypoplasia in association with VSD (depends upon the size of VSD)
- TA is classified as either VSD or TGA is absent or present. In one-fourth of the patients, there is a TGA

CLINICAL MANIFESTATIONS

- Cyanosis is usually severe from birth.
- Tachypnea and poor feeding usually manifest.
- Infants suffering from this condition usually present with a history of hypoxic spells.
- Cyanosis may be either with or without clubbing
- The second heart sound is single.
- A holosystolic (or early systolic) murmur of VSD is usually present at the lower left sternal border. A continuous murmur of PDA is present occasionally.

Tricuspid Atresia

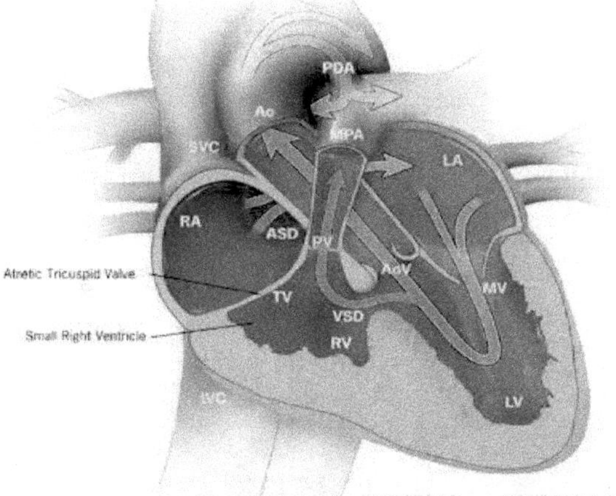

RA. Right Atrium
RV. Right Ventricle
LA. Left Atrium
LV. Left Ventricle

TV. Tricuspid Valve
MV. Mitral Valve
AoV. Aortic Valve
PV. Pulmonary Valve

MPA. Main Pulmonary Atery
Ao. Aorta
SVC. Superior Vena Cava
IVC. Inferior Vena Cava

ASD. Atrial Septal Defect
VSD. Ventricular Septal Defect
PDA.Patent Ductus Arteriosis

Normal Heart

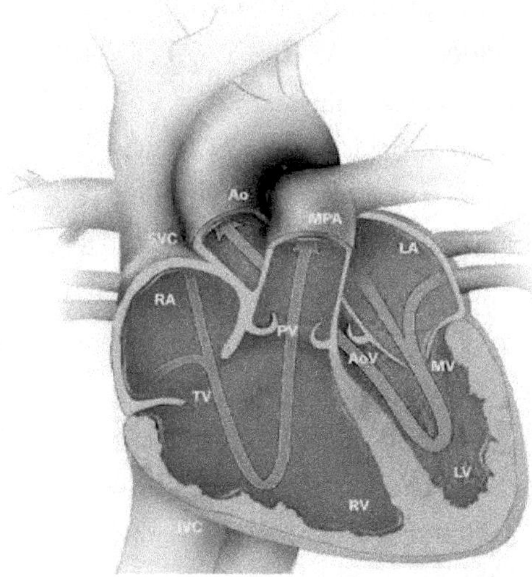

Electrocardiography

1. A notable finding of the TGA is the "Superior" QRS axis (between 0 and –90 degrees). But The superior QRS axis is present in only 50% of patients with TGA, and it may be found in the healthy population as well.

2. LVH is usually present; RAH or bi-atrial hypertrophy (BAH) is common.

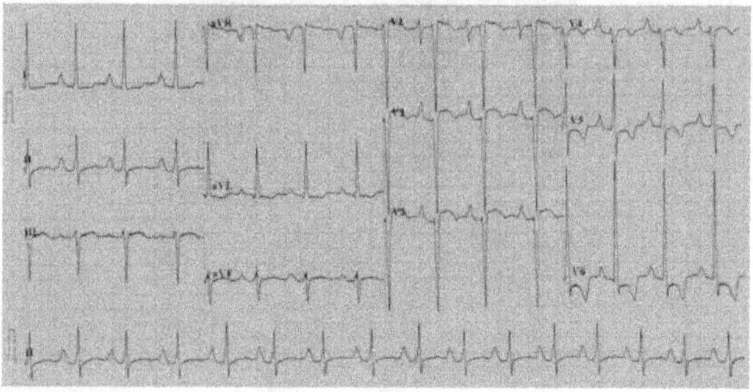

Total anomalous pulmonary venous connection:

- The frequency of TAPVC is 1% of all CHD.
- The pulmonary veins and the Left atrium are not connected directly with each other.
- The pulmonary veins connect either to the right atrium or to the great veins (SVC or IVC).
- Atrial communication is necessary to maintain life.
- Both oxygenated and deoxygenated blood get mixed In the right atrium, and the mixture is then distributed to other cardiac chambers.
- On cardiac catheterization, the oxygen saturation is found characteristically the same in all cardiac chambers

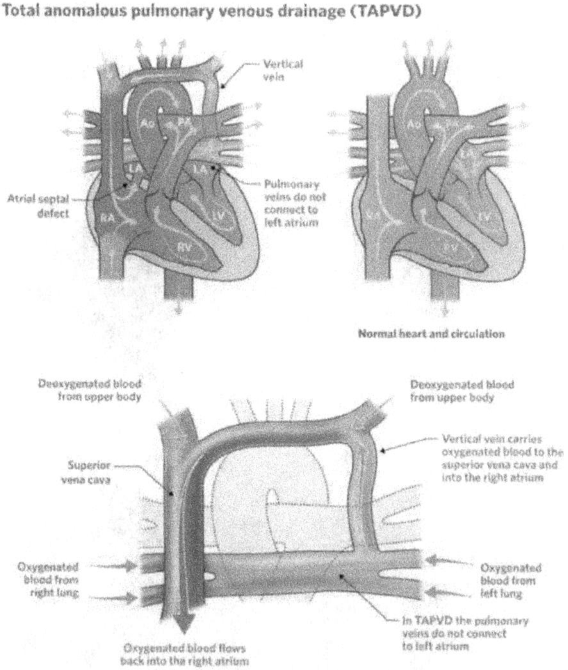

•

Anatomically there are four different types of TAPVC:

- Supracardiac is the most common type. A vertical vein connects the pulmonary veins to the innominate vein and SVC.
- Cardiac: The pulmonary veins connect either to coronary sinus or forms a connection with the right atrium.
- Infracardiac: A common pulmonary vein traverses the diaphragm and connects to the portal vein, ductus venosus, hepatic vein, or the IVC. The male population

is affected more than females for the infracardiac type (male/female ratio of 4:1).

- A mixed type is a combination of the above.

Total anomalous pulmonary venous return (classification)

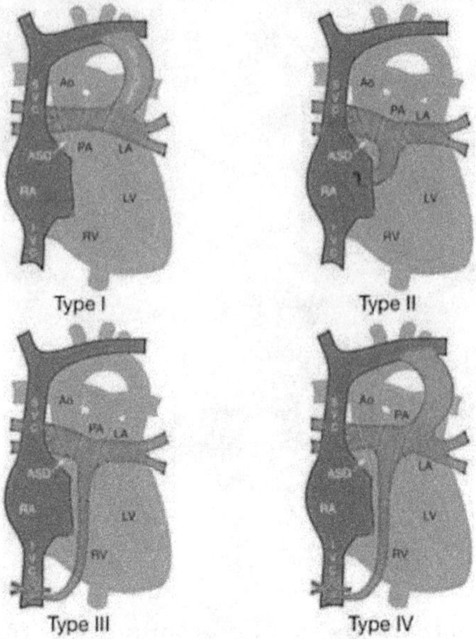

Physiologically, TAPVR can be categorized as

(i) obstructed, in which case the pulmonary venous return is impeded, which can lead to pulmonary venous hypertension and pulmonary edema.

(ii) unobstructed, in which case the anomalous drainage causes cyanosis due to mixing after return to the right side of the heart but does not cause respiratory distress in the first days after birth.

Clinical presentation:

- The clinical manifestations depend on either pulmonary venous connection obstruction is present or not.
- Frequent pulmonary infection, mild cyanosis, and CHF are the most common clinical presentations, even If there is no obstruction.
- Marked cyanosis, respiratory distress, and pulmonary congestion with pulmonary obstruction are characteristics findings.

Electrocardiography Findings:

- Without pulmonary venous obstruction, there is RVH of the so-called volume overload type (i.e., rsR′ in V1) and occasional RAH are present.
- If a pulmonary obstruction is present, there is RVH in the form of tall R waves in the right precordial leads and RAH is occasionally present

Note the presence of the right axis deviation, right atrial enlargement, and right ventricular hypertrophy in the following EKG.

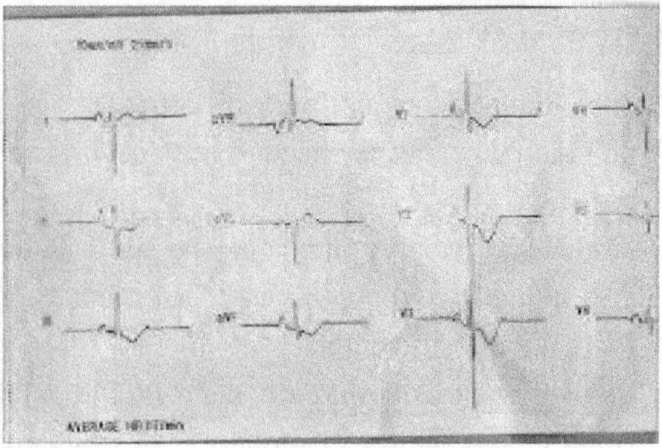

Persistent Truncus Arteriosus

- Persistent truncus arteriosus occurs in less than 1% of all congenital heart defects.
- Only a single arterial trunk with a unified truncal valve is present.
- This solitary trunk gives rise to pulmonary, systemic, and coronary circulations. A large perimembranous, infundibular VSD is present just below the truncus.
- The truncal valve it is often incompetent, Or it may be bicuspid, tricuspid, or quadricuspid, and

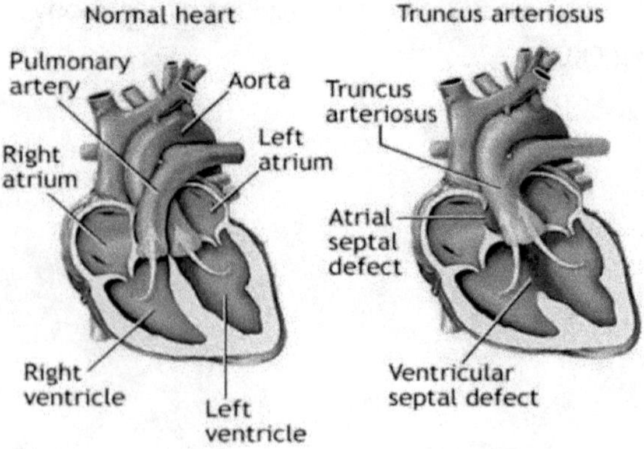

- This anomaly is divided into four types, according to Collett and Edwards' classification. The pulmonary blood flow is markedly increased in type I but decreased in type IV. In type II and III, it is almost normal.

Collett & Edwards classification of truncus arteriosus

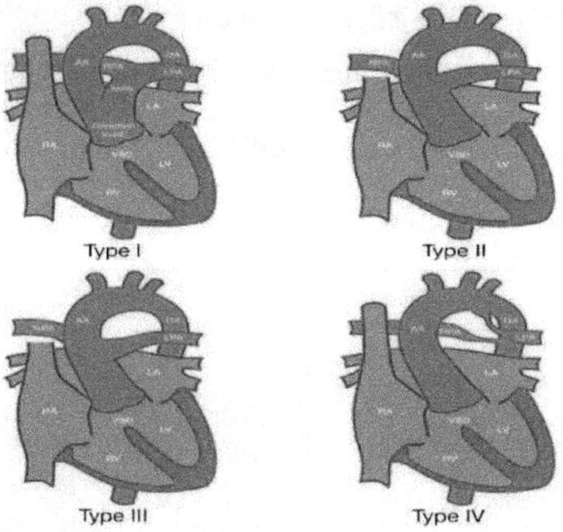

CLINICAL MANIFESTATIONS

- Cyanosis may be seen immediately after birth.
- Signs of congestive heart failure develop within several days to weeks after birth.
- There is a History of dyspnea while feeding.
- Failure to thrive and frequent respiratory infections are usually present in infants.
- The peripheral pulses are bounding, with wide pulse pressure.
- The second heart sound is single.

- Regurgitant systolic murmur Suggestive of VSD is usually audible along the left sternal border.

Electrocardiography

- The QRS axis is of +50 to +120 degrees. (normal)
- BVH is present in 70% of cases
- RVH or LVH is less common.
- Left atrial hypertrophy (LAH) is occasionally

Following ECG is showing biventricular hypertrophy.

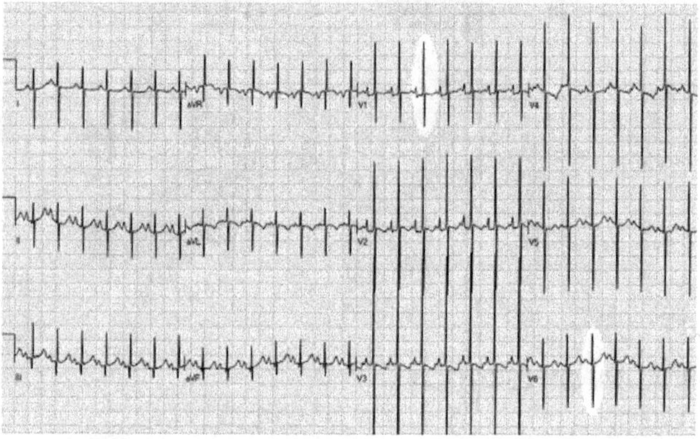

Complete transposition of great arteries

- D-TGA occurs in about 5% to 7% of all congenital heart defects.
- Males are affected more than females (male/female ratio of 3:1).
- In D-TGA, the aorta arises anteriorly from the right ventricle (RV) carrying desaturated blood to the body, and the pulmonary artery (PA) begins posteriorly from the left ventricle (LV) carrying oxygenated blood back to the lungs.

- Because the systemic and pulmonary circulations run side by side so, a connection between the two is necessary
- This connection is either with a ventricular septal defect (VSD), an atrial septal defect or at the great arterial level (patent ductus arteriosus).
- These connections allow systemic blood to go into the pulmonary circulation for oxygenation and oxygenated blood from the pulmonary circuit to enter the systemic circulation, to sustain life.
- VSD is present In almost half of patients with D-TGA and may be located anywhere in the ventricular septum.
- Most frequently associated congenital defect with TGA is patent foramen ovale (PFO) or a small PDA.

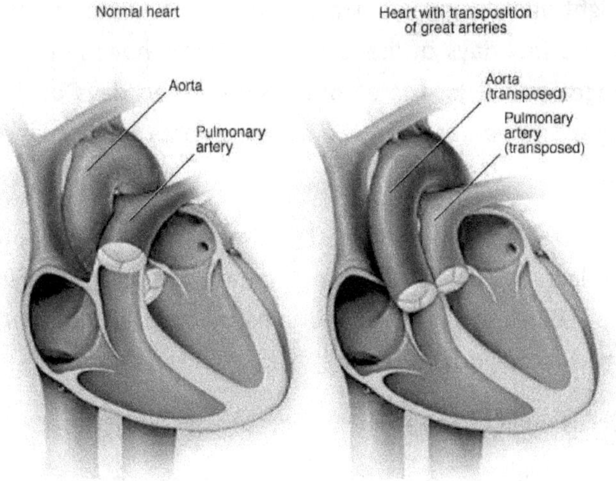

Clinical presentation:

- History of cyanosis from birth.
- Signs of congestive heart failure (CHF) with respiratory distress and feeding difficulties develop early during the newborn period.
- The single and loud second heart sound along with a holo-systolic murmur of VSD is present.
- Signs of symptoms of congestive heart failure may be present.
- In less than 1% of all patients with congenital heart defects, there is Congenitally Corrected Transposition of the Great Arteries (L-TGA)

Electrocardiography in D-TGA:

1. There is a rightward QRS axis deviation between +90 to +200 degrees.

2. Right ventricular hypertrophy (RVH) usually persists after the first few days of life. Some newborns have normal QRS voltages and QRS axis at birth. After three days of life, an upright T wave in V1 may be the only abnormality suggestive of RVH.

3. Biventricular hypertrophy (BVH) may be present in patients with large VSD, PDA, or pulmonary vascular obstructive disease because all these conditions produce an additional left ventricular hypertrophy (LVH).

4. Occasionally right atrial hypertrophy (RAH) is present.

Following is the ECG of a neonate with TGA with intact ventricular septum demonstrating right-axis deviation and prominent R waves in right chest leads and increased S waves in the left chest leads suggestive of RV hypertrophy.

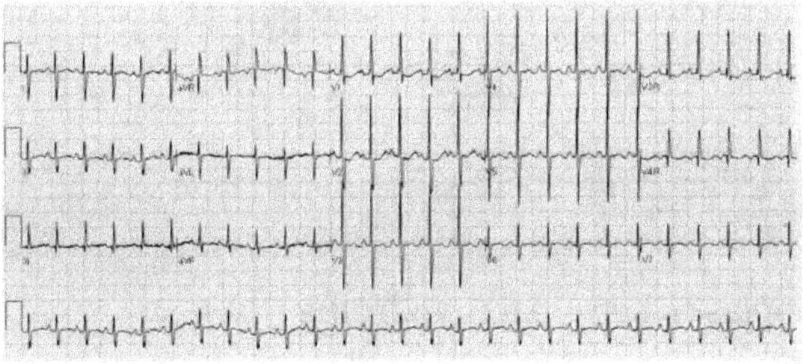

Electrocardiography in L-TGA:

1. the presence of Q waves in V4R or V1 or The absence of Q waves in V5 and V6 is characteristic of the condition. This occurs as the direction of ventricular septal depolarization is from the embryonic LV to RV.

2. Varying degrees of AV block is common. In about 50% of patients, First-degree AV block is present. Second-degree AV block may progress to third-degree AV-block. (complete heart block)

3. Occasionally Atrial arrhythmias and Wolff-Parkinson-White (WPW) preexcitation are present.

4. In a few complicated cases, either Atrial or ventricular hypertrophy, or both, may be present

Following is the ECG of a 4-year-old child with l-transposition of the great vessels. Note the absence of Q-waves in the left lateral precordial leads. Deep Q-waves are seen in the inferior leads.

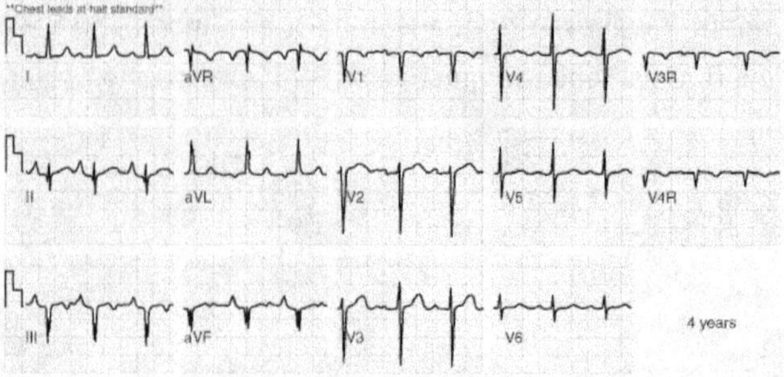

Hypoplastic Left Heart Syndrome

The prevalence of HLHS is 1% of all congenital heart defects.

This congenital defect is characterized by

- Left ventricular hypoplasia.
- Either the aortic or mitral valves or both may have atresia or critical stenosis.
- The ascending aorta and aortic arch are hypoplastic.
- The LV is small and nonfunctional or completely atretic.
- To supply blood to neck vessels and coronary arteries, PDA plays an essential role, as it provides blood in a retrograde direction to the transverse and ascending aorta
- The patient may have ASD (15%), or The atrial septum may be intact with a normal foramen ovale
- In about 10% of patients, A VSD appears
- COA is frequently an associated finding (up to 75%).
- up to 29% of cases brain abnormalities have been reported

Both pulmonary and systemic venous blood get thoroughly mix in the RA, and both systemic and pulmonary vessels received the same blood from RV.

Pulmonary resistance falls in the first few days of life.there is a net increase in blood flow towards the lungs, causing pulmonary congestion.on the other hand, reduced systemic flow causes tissue hypoxemia, metabolic acidosis, shock, or death in severe untreated cases.

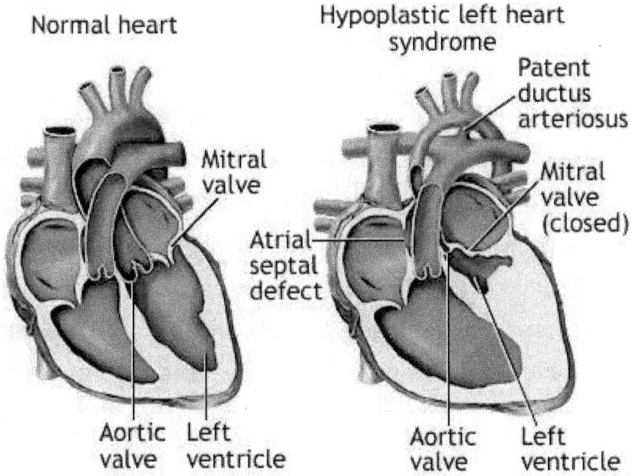

CLINICAL MANIFESTATIONS

- A neonate born with HLHS becomes critically ill within the first few hours to the early few days of life.
- The characteristic findings areTachycardia, dyspnea, pulmonary crackles, weak peripheral pulses, and vasoconstriction in extremities.

- Severe cyanosis may not be evident, but the patient might have a grayish-blue skin color due to poor perfusion.
- A heart murmur is usually absent
- Due to pulmonary hypertension, the second heart sound is loud and single.
- Hepatomegaly and gallop rhythm may develop in the case of CHF.

Echocardiography Findings:

- The ECG is almost always of RVH.
- Rarely, the ECG suggests LVH. Large R waves may be recorded in V5 and V6 because these leads record over the dilated RV, not over the hypoplastic LV.
- Sometimes ECG shows myocardial ischemic changes.
- Prolong PR interval, a broader QRS complex, decreased left-sided forces, an absence of septal Q waves in the inferior and lateral leads represent right-sided dominance.
- It is normal in 20%of individuals.

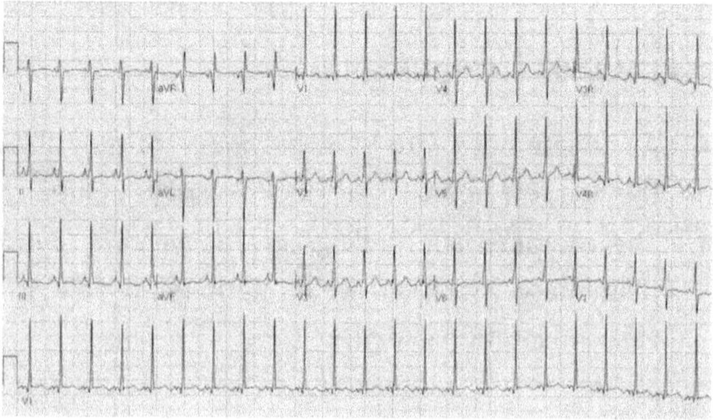

Ebstein's Anomaly

- Ebstein's anomaly of the tricuspid valve
- Its frequency is less than 1% of all congenital heart defects.
- The leaflets of the tricuspid valve(septal and posterior)are downward displaced into the RV cavity.
- So that a portion of the RV becomes the part of the RA, known as atrialized RV and functional hypoplasia of the RV results in Tricuspid regurgitation.
- PS, TOF, pulmonary atresia, or VSD are also associated with Ebstein anomaly.
- An interatrial communication (e.g., PFO, ASD) with a right-to-left shunt is present in all patients.
- WPW preexcitation is frequently associated with this anomaly and leads the patient to SVT.

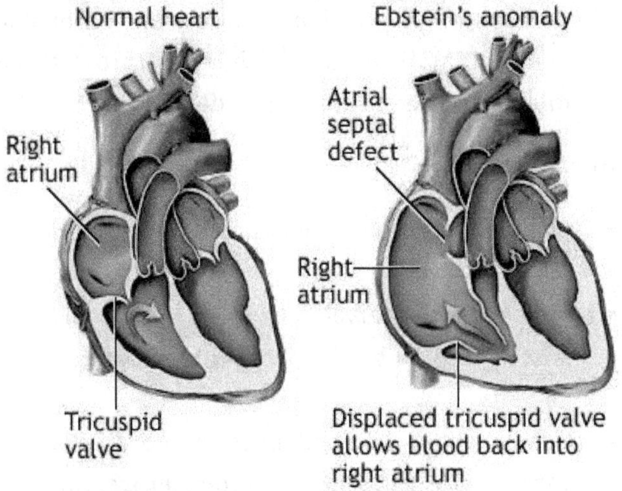

Clinical presentation:

- During the first few days of life, cyanosis and CHF develop in severe cases.
- Children with milder cases may complain of shortness of breath, fatigue, cyanosis, or palpitation on exertion.
- Mild to severe cyanosis is present
- in older infants and children, there is Clubbing of the fingers and toes.
- Cyanosis usually improves as pulmonary vascular resistance drops.
- Characteristic triple or quadruple rhythm is audible.
- At the left lower sternal border, a holosystolic murmur is audible due to tricuspid insufficiency
- Hepatomegaly is usually present.
- Patients with Ebstein anomaly carry a risk of stroke because of potential paradoxical embolism due to intermittent right to left shunting across a patent foramen ovale or Atrial septal defect.

Electrocardiography

- Characteristic ECG findings are RBBB and RAH.
- tall and broad P waves
- prolonged PR interval
- First-degree AV block is frequent, occurring in 40% of patients.
- Due to abnormal conduction in the atrialised right ventricle, a Fragmented QRS complex is formed.

- A WPW pattern of preexcitation syndrome is present in 15% to 20% of patients with occasional episodes of SVT.
- Tachyarrhythmias are due to accessory pathways usually present around the malformed TV.

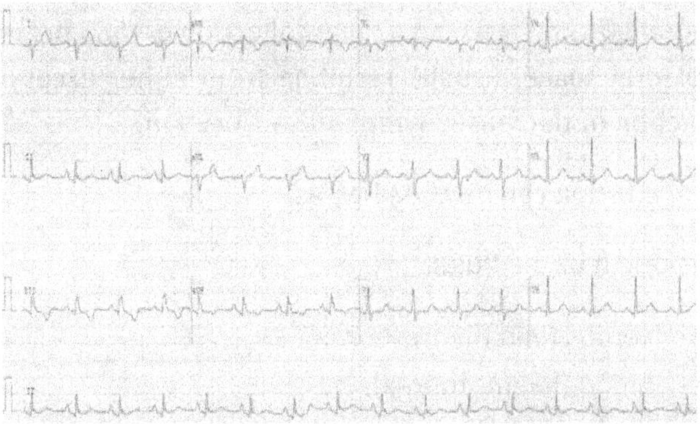

ECG in Ebstein's anomaly of the tricuspid valve showing right axis deviation of QRS, notched R waves in II, III, aVF, and V1 suggesting fragmented QRS. Peaked P waves indicate a right atrial abnormality

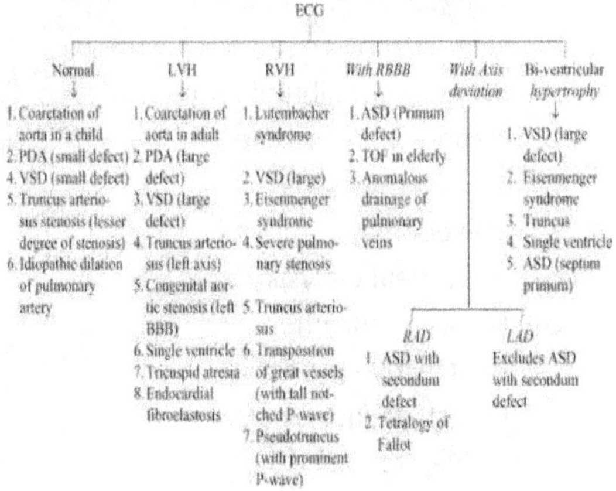

CHAPTER 18:
ECG changes in different medical conditions

Pleural effusion

A pleural effusion is a c abnormal collection of fluid present in the pleural space, usually resulting from either excess fluid production or decreased lymphatic absorption.

Pleural effusion can be classified as,

By the origin of the fluid:

- Serous fluid (hydrothorax)
- Blood (haemothorax)
- Chyle (chylothorax)
- Pus (pyothorax or empyema)

By pathophysiology:

- Transudative pleural effusion
    - Congestive heart failure
    - Liver cirrhosis
    - Severe hypoalbuminemia
    - Nephrotic syndrome
    - Acute atelectasis
    - Myxedema
    - Peritoneal dialysis
    - Meigs' syndrome
    - Obstructive uropathy
    - End-stage kidney disease
    - Exudative

- Exudative pleural effusion
    - Parapneumonic effusion due to pneumonia
    - Malignancy (either lung cancer or metastases to the pleura from elsewhere)
    - Infection (empyema due to bacterial pneumonia)
    - Trauma
    - Pulmonary infarction
    - Pulmonary embolism
    - Autoimmune disorders
    - Pancreatitis
    - Ruptured esophagus (Boerhaave's syndrome)
    - Rheumatoid pleurisy
    - Drug-induced lupus

In the case of pleural effusion, the fluid pushes the heart away from the chest wall, and EKG leads. Primarily this is typically seen in a large left-sided pleural effusion. Fluid also alters the electrical conduction property; that's why on ECG following findings are observed.

Typical findings in ECG are:

- Low voltage qrs.
- Poor R wave or even q waves
- QRS axis shifts are due to actual anatomical / electrical shifts
- T wave inversion as in this patient (see ECG below)

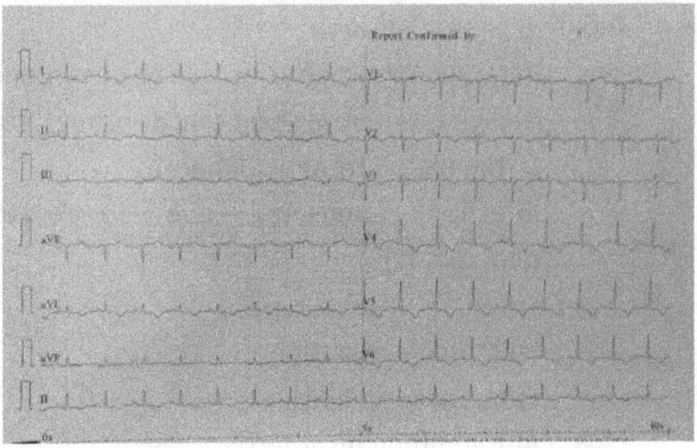

Sometimes extreme QRS axis deviation mimics acute myocardial infarction.

Pericardial Effusion

Pericardial effusion ("fluid around the heart"). It is an abnormal accumulation of fluid in the pericardial cavity.

In the pericardial cavity, limited space is available, and fluid accumulation leads to increased intrapericardial pressure. This pressure can negatively affect heart function. A pericardial effusion with enough pressure, which can adversely affect the functioning of the heart is called <u>cardiac tamponade</u>.

Causes:

- Pericarditis
- Viral infection (coxsackievirus)
- Infection including tuberculosis
- Drug-eluting stents
- Inflammatory disorders, such as lupus, rheumatoid arthritis, and post-myocardial infarction pericarditis (Dressler's syndrome)

- Cancer that has spread to the pericardium
- Trichinosis
- Kidney failure with excessive blood levels of urea nitrogen
- Minoxidil
- Hypothyroidism
- Heart surgery (Postpericardiotomy syndrome)

Pericardial fluid may be,

- transudative (congestive heart failure, myxoedema, nephrotic syndrome),
- exudative (tuberculosis, spread from empyema)
- hemorrhagic (trauma, rupture of aneurysms, malignant effusion).
- Malignant (due to fluid accumulation caused by metastasis)

Signs and symptoms:

pericardial effusion include the following medical presentations,

- Chest pain, pressure, discomfort
- Light-headedness, syncope
- Palpitations
- Cough
- Dyspnea
- Hoarseness
- Anxiety and confusion
- Hiccoughs

Examination findings in patients with pericardial effusion are:

- Classic Beck triad of pericardial tamponade is Hypotension, muffled heart sounds, jugular venous distention
- Pulsus paradoxus
- Pericardial friction rub
- Tachycardia
- Hepatojugular reflux
- Tachypnea
- Decreased breath sounds
- Dullness to percussion just beneath the angle of the left scapula is called Ewart sign.
- Hepatosplenomegaly
- Weakened peripheral pulses, edema, and cyanosis

ECG findings:

Classically, the electrocardiographic changes of acute pericarditis progress through 4 progressive stages:

- Stage I - ST-segment elevation and PR-segment depression in all leads.
- Stage II - The ST and PR segments become normal.
- Stage III - Widespread T-wave inversions. (This is important to differentiate it from myocardial infarction as T-wave inversions in pericarditis usually occur after ST-segment normalization, unlike myocardial infarction)
- Stage IV – The T-waves become normal again.

- There are no typical electrocardiographic abnormalities in the Patients with uremic pericarditis.

Low-voltage QRS complexes, classically defined as the total amplitude of the QRS complex less than 0.5 mv in the limb leads and <1 mv in the precordial leads, can also be seen in large effusions and tamponade

Pericarditis:

inflammation of the pericardial membrane is defined as pericarditis. It is clinically present as sharp chest pain. The pain is characterized by sudden onset, radiation to the shoulders, neck, or back. It typically gets better while sitting up and worsen by lying down or deep breathing. Other symptoms could be fever, weakness, palpitations, and shortness of breath. Occasionally these symptoms may appear gradually.

A friction rub is a classic sign of pericarditis, best heard at the lower left sternal border, with a stethoscope. The patient might have diaphoresis (excessive sweating); possibility of heart failure in the form of pericardial tamponade resulting in pulses paradoxus, and the Beck's triad of low blood pressure (due to decreased cardiac output), distant (muffled) heart sounds, and jugular venous distension(raised JVP).

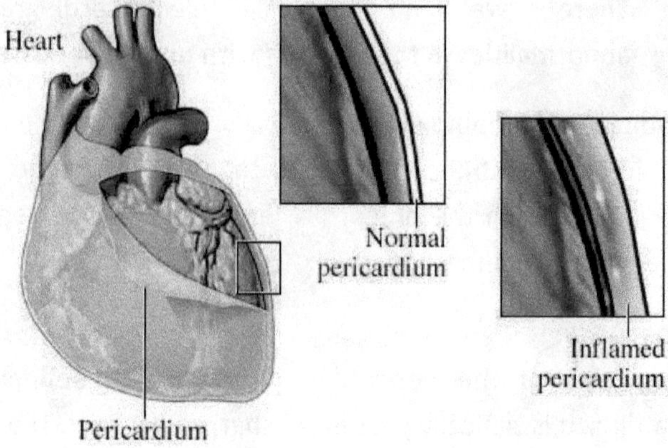

Specific causes of pericarditis include the following:

- Idiopathic causes
- Infectious conditions, such as viral, bacterial, and mycobacterium tuberculous.
- Inflammatory disorders, such as scleroderma, RA, SLE, and rheumatic fever
- Metabolic diseases, such as hypothyroidism and renal failure.
- Cardiovascular diseases, such as acute MI, Dressler syndrome, and aortic dissection
- Miscellaneous causes, such as neoplasms, drugs, irradiation, cardiovascular procedures, and trauma

ECG CHANGES:

ECG can be diagnostic in acute pericarditis and typically shows diffuse ST elevation.

- ST-segment elevations in all leads, except in lead aVR and V1.

- PR-segment depression possible in any lead, except in lead aVR (seen in 80% of patients with viral pericarditis)
- sinus tachycardia
- In the case of subclinical pericardial effusion, low voltage QRS -complexes are also seen.
- The PR depression is often early presentation as the thin atria are affected more quickly than the ventricles during pericarditis.

ECG changes can be classified into four phases according to the tie period and T-waves morphology in ECG

- Stage 1 is observed after the onset of acute pain. T waves are upright in all leads. It lasts up to hours and days.
- Stage 2 of the disease occurs several days after the acute attack. ST-segment returns to baseline, followed by flattening of the T waves. This stage lasts up to a few weeks.
- T waves become inverted in stage 3 but no Q wave formation.
- In stage 4, the ECG returns to the standard, weeks to months after the initial onset. The T-wave inversion may persist indefinitely in the chronic inflammatory conditions.

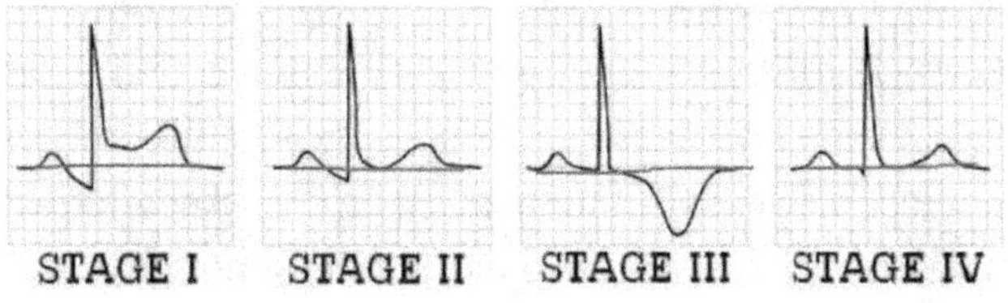

In the figure above, the blue line is representing the ECG baseline.

One of the most life-threatening complications of pericarditis is cardiac tamponade. It is a condition in which so much fluid is accumulated between heart and pericardium leading to compression and malfunction of the heart. This results in heart failure.

Cardiomyopathies

Cardio stands for cardiac or heart, Myo stands for Muscles, and pathy stands for Pathology or disease. So cardiomyopathy is the group of disorders in which heart muscles are affected. They are weak and unable to perform properly. Cardiomyopathies could be acquired or inherited.

Main types of cardiomyopathies are,

- Hypertrophic cardiomyopathy
- Restrictive cardiomyopathy
- Dilated cardiomyopathy
- Arrhythmogenic right ventricular dysplasia
- Transthyretin amyloid cardiomyopathy (ATTR-CM)

Hypertrophic cardiomyopathy:

In hypertrophic cardiomyopathy (HCM), there is left ventricular hypertrophy (LVH), occurring without any apparent cause like hypertension or aortic stenosis. LVH could be mild to severe. In mild hypertrophy, muscle thickness is 13-15 mm, and in extreme myocardial thickening, muscle thickness of 30-60 mm may be seen. But in most cases, it is characteristically asymmetric with more involvement of the ventricular septum.

It is primarily a genetic disorder with autosomal dominant inheritance.

Patients may have recurrent exertional dyspnea, chest pain, or syncope. In young athletes, It is the number one cause of sudden cardiac death. Annual mortality is estimated at 1-2 %.

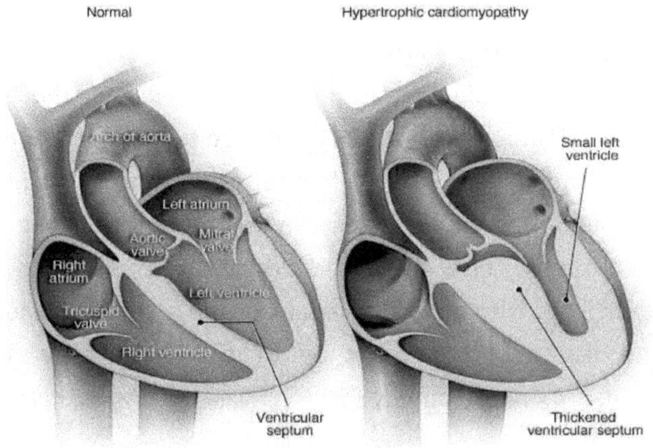

Electrocardiographic Features are as following:

- Left atrial enlargement
- Left ventricular hypertrophy with associated ST-segment / T-wave abnormalities
- Deep, narrow ("dagger-like") Q waves in the lateral leads
- Giant precordial T-wave inversions (strain pattern)
- Signs of WPW (short PR, delta wave).
- Dysrhythmias: atrial fibrillation, supraventricular tachycardias, PACs, PVCs, VT

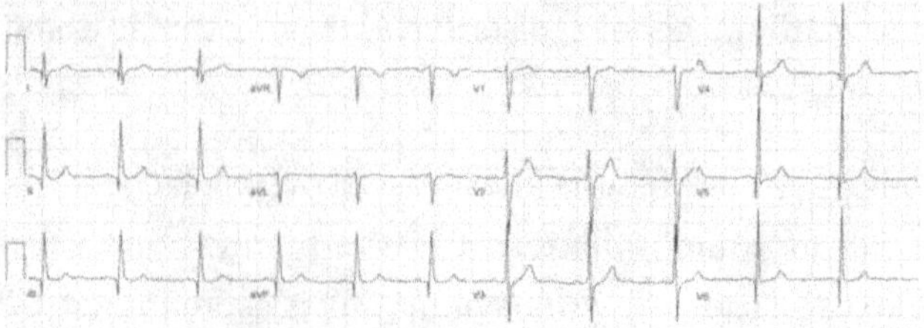

ECG with dagger Q-waves.

Restrictive cardiomyopathy

In Restrictive cardiomyopathy (RCM), the walls of the heart become stiff and less elastic as compared to healthy tissue but not thickened (like in HCM). Thus the heart is prevented from stretching during the cardiac cycle, and there is no filling with blood properly. There is reduced diastolic filling of one or both ventricles but with normal or near-normal systolic function. It is the least common subtype of cardiomyopathy. RCM accounts for approximately 5% only.

Symptoms may include the following:

- Gradually worsening shortness of breath
- Progressive exercise intolerance
- Orthopnea and Fatigue
- Weight loss and loss of appetite.
- Paroxysmal nocturnal dyspnea
- Abdominal discomfort or liver tenderness
- Chest pain, primarily in patients with amyloidosis or due to angina
- Palpitations

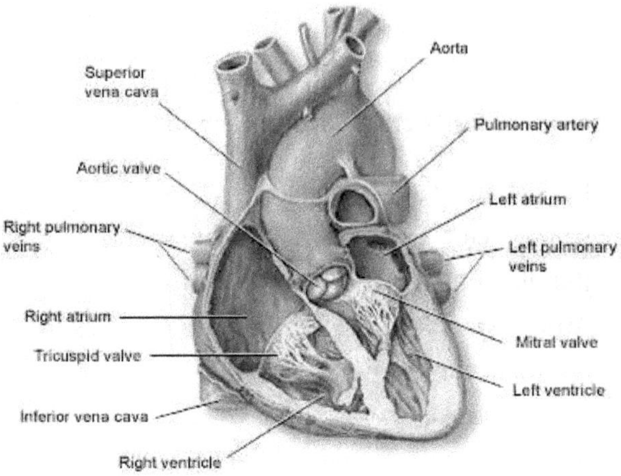

On examination:

- Increased jugular venous pressure
- Decreased pulse volume
- Regular S 1 and S 2 but Loud early diastolic filling sound (S 3)
- Un-significant Murmurs due to mitral and tricuspid valve regurgitation

Causes:

- Hemochromatosis. (deposition of iron in heart tissue)
- Sarcoidosis. (abnormal immune response causes tiny lumps of cells in the body's organs, including the heart.)
- Amyloidosis. (abnormal proteins deposition in the body's organs, including the heart.)
- Connective tissue disorders

- Specific cancer treatments, such as radiation and chemotherapy

ECG Features of Restrictive Cardiomyopathy

- Low voltage QRS complexes
- Non-specific ST-segment / T wave changes
- Bundle branch blocks
- Atrioventricular block (3rd degree AV block may occur in sarcoidosis)
- Pathological Q waves
- Atrial and ventricular dysrhythmias (74% of patients have atrial fibrillation)

Following is the ECG recording from a patient with amyloid infiltration of the heart. there is low voltage in the precordial leads and a prolonged PR interval.

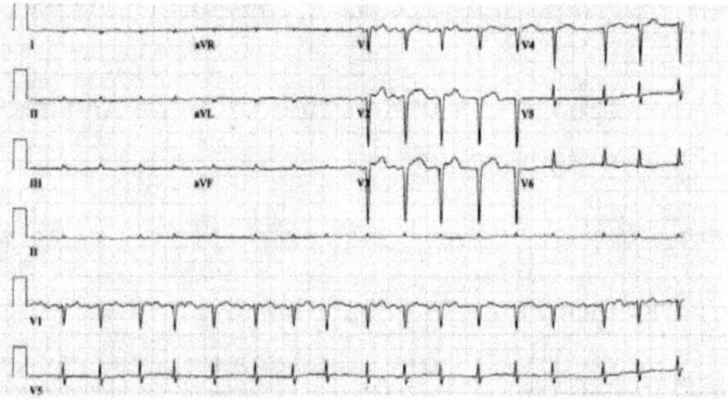

Dilated cardiomyopathy

Dilated cardiomyopathy is a progressive disorder of heart muscle that is characterized by left ventricular enlargement and its ability to contract during systole. The right ventricle also become dilated and dysfunctional over time.

Signs and Symptoms:

- Dyspnea on exertion, shortness of breath, cough
- Fatigue
- Orthopnea
- paroxysmal nocturnal dyspnea
- Increasing edema, weight, or abdominal circumference

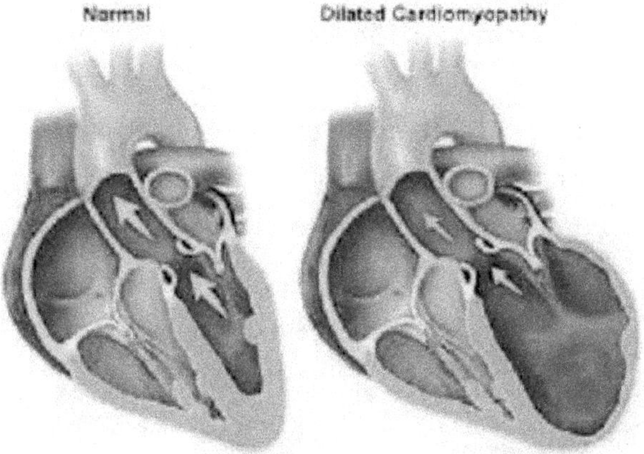

On physical examination, there are signs of heart failure (Tachypnea, Tachycardia, Hypertension or hypotension) there could be

- Pulmonary edema (crackles and wheezes)
- Signs of hypoxia (e.g., cyanosis, clubbing)
- Jugular venous distension (JVD)
- S3 gallop
- Enlarged liver
- Peripheral edema

The apical impulse is generally within 10 cm of the midsternal line. In a person with dilated cardiomyopathy, the apex beat will be shifted towards the axilla.

Causes:

- Medical conditions like Coronary heart disease, high blood pressure, diabetes, thyroid disease, viral hepatitis and HIV
- Infections, especially viral infections (causes inflammation of the heart muscle)
- Alcohol
- During the last month of pregnancy
- within 5 months after giving birth.
- Certain toxins such as cobalt
- Certain drugs (such as cocaine and amphetamines)
- Chemotherapeutic drugs (doxorubicin and daunorubicin)

ECG changes:

ECG is an essential tool to differentiate between heart failure due to MI and dilated cardiac myopathy

- left ventricular enlargement
- Atrial fibrillation or premature ventricular complexes.
- Conduction delay mainly left bundle-branch block
- Varying degrees of the atrioventricular block is noted.
- An ECG showing atrial fibrillation increases the likelihood of heart failure.

Arrhythmogenic right ventricular dysplasia

Arrhythmogenic right ventricular dysplasia (ARVD) is a sporadic type of cardiomyopathy. It occurs when the heart muscle tissue of the right ventricle dies and is replaced by scar tissue. This disrupts the heart's electrical conduction pathway and signals, causing arrhythmias. It is known as Right ventricular cardiomyopathy or Right ventricular dysplasia. The cause is unknown but might occur due to genetic factors. More prevalent among Young adults. More common in males than females. There are no definite presenting symptoms, but there is a history of sudden cardiac death in the family.

ECG changes :

- Epsilon wave (most specific)
- T wave inversion in V1-3
- Prolonged S-wave upstroke
- QRS widening in V1-3
- ventricular tachycardia with LBBB.

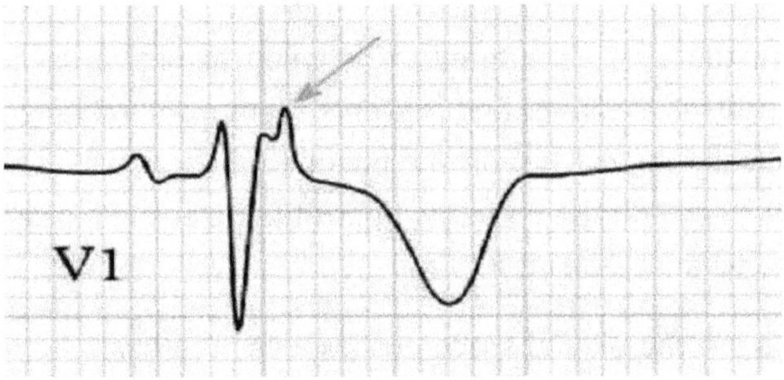

Transthyretin amyloid cardiomyopathy (ATTR-CM)

In this disease, there is the deposition of transthyretin amyloid fibrils in the heart. The left ventricle stiffens and doesn't relax in diastole. It is a life-threatening, progressive, infiltrative disease. It commonly presents with symptoms of heart failure or arrhythmias. As it is an infiltrative disease, it affects other systems of the body as well.

ECG findings:

- LOW voltage complexes in all leads
- Pseudo-infarct pattern
- Atrial fibrillation and flutter
- Intraventricular conduction delay

Low-voltage complexes on ECG and increased mass on echocardiography are the best diagnostic tests of infiltrative cardiomyopathy.

On Cardiac Holter monitoring there is a lack of heart rate variability due to autonomic dysfunction

Pneumothorax

Pneumo means air and thorax stands for thoracic cavity

When the air gets entered in between to pleural layers, it compresses the lungs and prevents them from inflating. This results in lung collapse. If the pneumothorax is significant, it shifts the mediastinum to the opposite side and compromises hemodynamic stability.

The air in the pleural space pushes away the heart from the chest wall and, since air is a poor conductor of electricity, it makes the waveforms on the EKG smaller.

Tension pneumothorax is responsible for causing true ischemic changes in ECG along with PR-segment elevation in the inferior leads and PR-segment depression in the aVR lead.

Left pneumothorax was associated with ECG features such as low QRS voltage in the limb leads and precordial leads, reduced R-wave progression in the precordial leads, and an increased QRS complex (QRS) voltage ratio (aVF/I). while right pneumothorax caused no ECG changes, but some studies suggest that the right-sided pneumothorax can be caused by reduced R wave progression in the precordial leads too.

All of these changes are reversible after the improvement of pneumothorax.

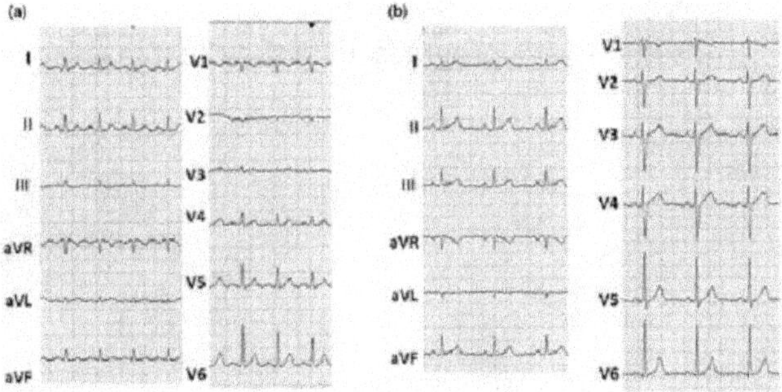

A=ECG with pneumothorax, low voltage complexes in lead II and III.

B=ECG after improvement

Dextrocardia

Dextrocardia is a heart defect by birth In which the heart is on the right side instead of the left side of the chest. As ECG leads are routinely placed on the left side, the distance between heart and chest leads becomes increased. The EKG shows decreased waveform voltages as the leads headway from lead V1 to V6. Usually, the leads were placed on the left side of the patient's chest, lead V2 is further from the heart than V1, and V3 is further than V2, and so on. V6 is the furthest from the heart and therefore exhibits the lowest voltage of all. The P wave direction in the frontal plane points unusually to the patient's right side (+135 degrees) and strengthens the suspicion of Dextrocardia.

- Right axis deviation
- Positive QRS complexes in lead aVR
- inversion of all complexes in lead I
- Absent R-wave progression in the chest leads

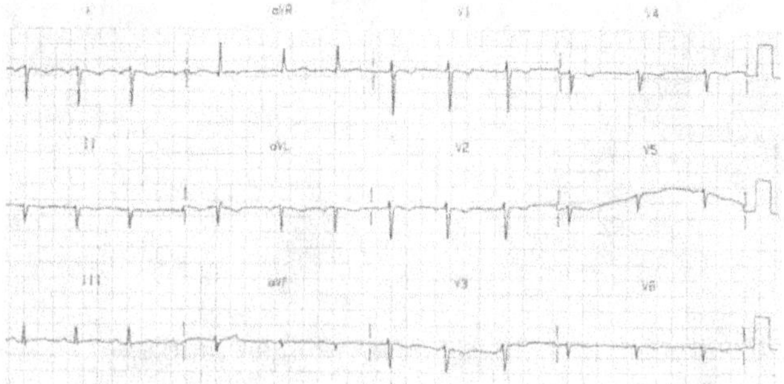

COPD (Chronic obstructive pulmonary diseases)

among older adults, Chronic obstructive pulmonary disease (COPD) is a prevalent lung disease

Among different causes of low voltage ECG, it is the most frequent one. In COPD, Diseased airways trap excessive air in the lungs. As air is a poor conductor of electrical current, and so the voltage of some or all leads on the EKG is lowered. Hypoxia or low oxygen level in the blood is another common cause of increased heart rate (sinus tachycardia). But in severe or long-standing cases, it may lead to bradycardia, that is why all patients who are on ventilator support or those with chronic lung disease if presents with sudden bradycardia should be evaluated carefully for hypoxia.

Similarly, Patients with COPD are usually treated with sympathetic agonists to improve respiratory symptoms, which may lead to sinus tachycardia as a side effect of sinus bradycardia in case of profound use.

Typical ECG Findings in COPD

1. The most typical ECG findings in case of emphysema are:

- The right shift of the P wave axis
- P waves in the inferior leads are prominent
- P waves in leads I and aVL are flattened or inverted
- The right shift of the QRS axis towards +90 degrees
- PR and ST segments that "sag" or dips below the baseline due to exaggerated atrial depolarization.
- Low voltage QRS complexes

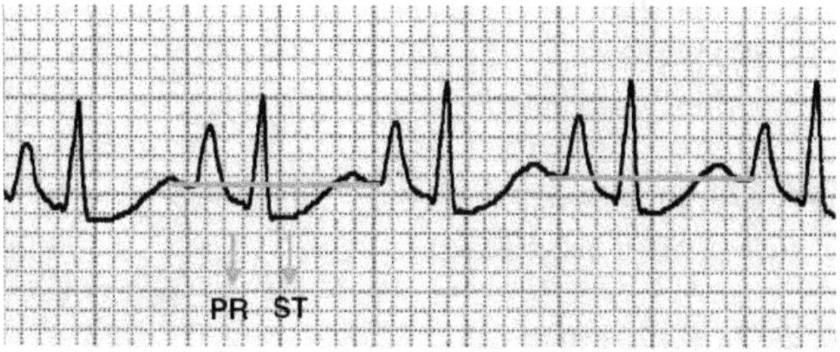

Sagging of the PR and ST segments below the baseline

2. With the development of cor pulmonale

- Right atrial enlargement (P pulmonale)
- Right ventricular hypertrophy

3. Other ECG changes that may be seen

- Right bundle branch block (usually due to RVH)
    - Multifocal atrial tachycardia

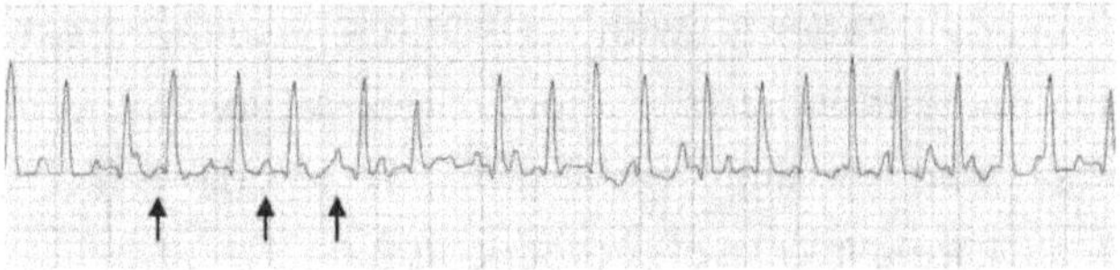

irregular, rapid and narrow-complex with at least three different P-wave morphologies (arrows)

Athlete's Heart

The assessment of the athlete's heart is always challenging for the Physician. Many of the EKG changes and dysrhythmias, which are related to an athlete's heart, are considered abnormal in a healthy population.

- Sinus bradycardia
- sinus arrhythmia
- sinus pause
- escape beats
- various AV blocks

above mentioned are few of the examples of dysrhythmias often experienced by an athlete.

On the EKG

- changes in the P wave and QRS complex are very common.
- Increased P wave voltage (signifying left or right atrial enlargement0
- increased QRS voltage (representing right or left ventricular hypertrophy)
- ECG reveals junctional rhythm and right intraventricular conduction delay (RSR in V1).

Effects of Cancer on the EKG

Malignant carcinomas and some anti-cancer drugs directly affect the heart and cause particular changes on the electrocardiogram.

Following are the manifestations of malignant invasion of the heart by carcinomas

- Pericardial Effusion
- cardiac tamponade
- increased heart size
- heart failure
- new heart murmurs

Other manifestations are,

- Radiation therapy may lead to pericarditis.
- Chemotherapy can cause acute or chronic systolic heart failure
- Hypercoagulable states can lead to pulmonary embolism.
- Metastatic disease may result in significant electrolyte disturbances.

- Obstructive or chemotherapy-induced renal failure may cause hyperkalemia
- Cancer patients may suffer from hypovolemic due to nausea and vomiting or bleeding.
- Metastatic spread to the bone may be associated with increase serum calcium levels

Effects of Stroke on the EKG

Subarachnoid hemorrhage is typically associated with repolarization abnormalities on the EKG. These findings are

- deep, symmetrically inverted T waves in the V leads
- to a prolonged QT interval.

Raised ICP is associated with specific distinctive ECG changes:

- Widespread giant T-wave inversions also are known as "cerebral T waves."
- QT prolongation.
- Bradycardia due to the Cushing reflex

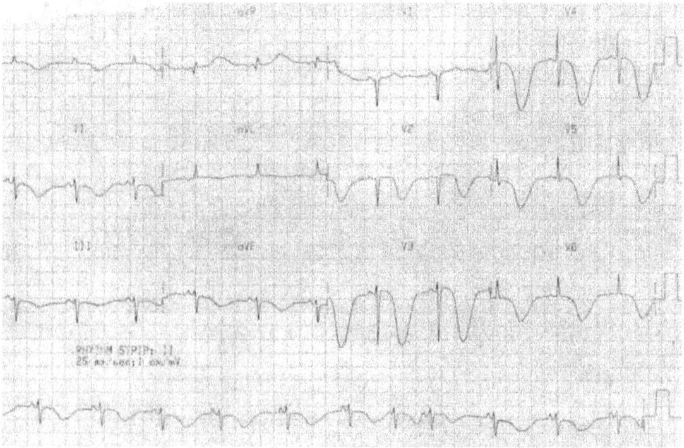

Neonatal SLE

Neonatal lupus erythematosus is a disease characterized by the appearance of the systemic lupus erythematosus (SLE) symptoms in a newborn from a mother with SLE. Neonatal SLE most commonly presents with a rash resembling subacute cutaneous lupus erythematosus, and sometimes with other systemic abnormalities such as complete heart block or hepatosplenomegaly.

Some infants might have no skin lesions at birth but sometimes develop them during the first weeks of life. Neonatal lupus is usually benign and has a self-limited course.

It is related to the mothers who carry the Anti-SSA/Ro antibodies, which is associated strongly with the subacute cutaneous lupus erythematosus form of the disease.

Low heart rate (bradycardia) is generally the main clinical presentation that leads to the diagnosis. It is described as the disorder of the electrical conduction system within the heart muscle. Newborn kids with a heart rate lower than 55 bpm have a poor prognosis and outcome and higher chance to need pace-maker implantation. Kids with congenital heart block have a higher incidence of health-related issues like infections than other kids.

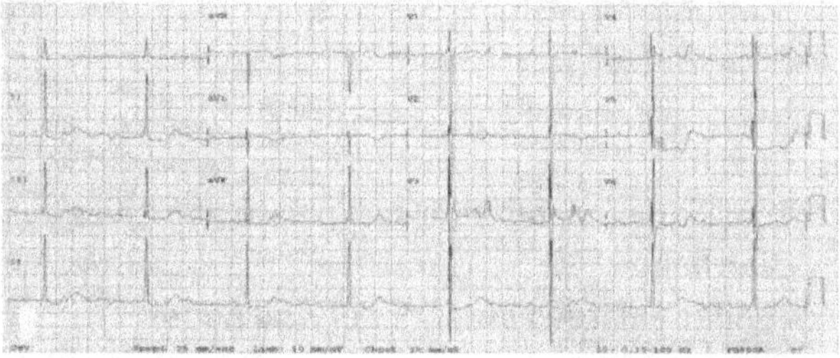

ECG is showing a complete heart block with a ventricular rate of 43/min.

Acute Rheumatic Fever (ARF)

Acute rheumatic fever (ARF) is best described as an inflammation of the heart but also involving skin, joints, and brain. It develops after infection with Group A streptococci, such as "strep" throat or scarlet fever. This disease is one of the most important causes of cardiovascular morbidity and mortality in developing countries.

Pathology

Pharyngeal infection of Group A streptococcal (GAS) infection is the most frequent triggering cause of rheumatic fever. In ARF, antibodies against the M antigen protein found in the streptococcal cell wall cross-react with cardiac myosin causing carditis. Proper antibiotic treatment of streptococcal pharyngitis prevents acute rheumatic fever in most cases.

Features suggestive of GAS infection

- Characteristics indicative of viral infection
- Sudden onset sore throat with painful swallowing
- Conjunctivitis
- Fever
- Coryza
- Scarlet fever rash
- Hoarseness
- Headache, nausea, and vomiting
- Cough
- Tonsillar exudates with soft palate petechiae
- Diarrhea
- Tender enlarged anterior cervical nodes
- Characteristic exanthems

Patients age 5-15 years with a history of exposure.

Signs and symptoms of rheumatic fever include

- fever,
- migratory arthritis in large joints,
- abdominal pain,
- erythema marginatum (a ring-shaped rash located on the trunk and upper parts of arms and legs),
- Sydenham chorea,
- subcutaneous nodules,
- epistaxis,
- shortness of breath and chest pain.

Clinical diagnosis is made by using **Modified Jones Criteria**

Evidence of previous group A streptococcal pharyngitis is essential to diagnose rheumatic fever.

- The major diagnostic criteria include Carditis, polyarthritis, chorea, subcutaneous nodules, erythema marginatum

- The minor diagnostic criteria include Fever, polyarthralgia, prolonged PR interval, elevated peak erythrocyte sedimentation rate (ESR) and C-reactive protein (CRP)

ECG changes:

- On electrocardiography (ECG), sinus tachycardia is most commonly associated with acute rheumatic heart disease.
- First-degree atrioventricular (AV) block (prolongation of the PR interval) is observed in some patients

- Second-degree (intermittent) and third-degree (complete) AV block with progression to a ventricular standstill is also seen in few cases
- If acute rheumatic fever is associated with pericarditis, ST-segment elevation may be most evident in leads II, III, aVF, and V_4 -V_6.
- Patients with rheumatic heart disease may develop atrial flutter, multifocal atrial tachycardia, or atrial fibrillation due to chronic mitral valve disease

Adequate therapy for Group A streptococcus pharyngitis is essential for the prevention of rheumatic fever.

Penicillin V

- < 27 kg: 250 mg BID/TID
- >27 kg: 500 mg BID/TID
- Ten days

Amoxicillin

- 50 mg/kg daily
- Ten days

Benzathine Penicillin G

- <27 kg: 600,000 U IM
- >27 kg: 1.2 million U IM
- Once

In the case of penicillin allergy:

- Cephalexin/Cefadroxil for ten days
- Azithromycin ,12 mg/kg,daily for 5 days (max 500 mg)

- Clindamycin, 20 mg/kg in 3 divided doses (max 1.8 g/day) for 10 days

Due to repeated attacks of **acute rheumatic** fever, the heart valves get permanent damage, a condition known as rheumatic heart disease. Medical conditions like heart failure, infective endocarditis, and atrial fibrillation could occur due to these damaged valves.

Antibiotic prophylaxis should be given to patients with a documented history of ARF until the age of 21 or for a minimum of five years in case of no cardiac involvement. Patients with valvular abnormalities should receive prophylaxis for a whole life.

Infective Endocarditis

OVERVIEW

- endocarditis is a disease, characterized by inflammation of the endocardium
- It typically affects the heart valves and usually caused by infection
- the presentation can be acute, subacute or chronic
- most commonly affecting the aortic valve is the aortic valve, but in developing countries still, the mitral wall is the most frequently involved.
- the most common cause of fulminant endocarditis is *S. aureus*

- always be suspicious of endocarditis in patients with *S. aureus* septicemia.

CAUSE

Organisms

- *Staphylococcus aureus* (MSSA or MRSA)
- Coagulase-negative Staphylococci: *S. epidermidis, S. lugdenensis*
- *Streptococcus viridans*
- *Streptococcus Bovis*
- *Enterococcus*
- HACEK organisms

-> *Haemophilus aphrophilus, parainfluenza*, and *paraphrophilus*
-> *Actinobacillus actinomycetemcomitans*
-> *Cardiobacterium hominis*
-> *Eikenella corrodens*
-> *Kingella kingae*

- Fungi

Culture negative endocarditis

- *Brucella*
- *Bartonella*
- *Coxiella burnetti* (Q fever)

- *Chlamydia*
- *Legionella*
- *Mycoplasma*
- Whipple's disease (*Trophyerma whipplei*)

RISK FACTORS

Cardiac lesions

- congenital heart disease
- rheumatic heart disease
- mitral valve prolapse
- valve regurgitation
- degenerative valve disease
- prosthetic valve (1-5%) – early presentation in less than 60 days or late presentation in more than 60 days)

Predisposition to infection

- IV drug abusers.
- Hemodialysis
- High-risk surgery (e.g., dental, respiratory and infective)
- long lines
- bone marrow transplant recipients
- immunosuppressed (e.g., HIV)

CLINICAL FEATURES

History

- 50% of cases happen in patients with normal valves!
- spectrum:
  — asymptomatic
  — malaise, night sweats, anemia, weight loss
  — crashing cardiogenic shock and sepsis
- haematuria (glomerulonephritis)
- embolic complications
  — stroke (especially if PFO), intracranial hemorrhage
  — septic pulmonary emboli
  — splenic infarction
- presence of risk factors

EXAMINATION

- Skin rash
- Splinter hemorrhages
- conjunctival hemorrhages
- Oslers nodes (tender nodules on pulps of fingers and toes)
- Janeway lesions (non-tender hemorrhagic pulps on fingers and toes)
- Roth spots (retinal hemorrhages with a pale center)
- Splenomegaly

- New neurological signs
- New murmur, e.g., aortic regurgitation
- Left ventricular failure (basal crackles and effusions in lungs)
- Emboli — major arteries, pulmonary, spleen
- Haematuria

INVESTIGATIONS

Bedside

- **ECG: broadening of the PR interval, p mitrale, dysrhythmia**

Laboratory

- Blood cultures (positive in 90% of the cases.) — need at least two sets drawn 12 hours apart. — minimum of 3 out four sets positive with first and last positive set >1 hour apart
- Serology for causative organisms
- Rheumatoid factor
- if culture-negative, PCR for microbial 16S ribosomal RNA genes from valve tissue.

ECHO

Trans thorax echocardiography is 60% sensitive while Transoesophageal echocardiography is 90-99% sensitive and have a specificity of 90%

oscillating intracardiac mass observed

- on valves
- on supporting structures
- in the path of regurgitant jets,
- on implanted material
- in the absence of an alternative explanation
- abscess
- new partial dehiscence of prosthetic valve

DIAGNOSIS

Use the Modified Duke Criteria

- Two major criteria, or
- One major and three minor criteria, or
- Five minor criteria

Major criteria

Positive blood culture for Infective Endocarditis Typical microorganism consistent with IE from 2 separate blood cultures, as noted below:

— viridans streptococci, *Streptococcus bovis*, or HACEK group, or

—community-acquired *Staphylococcus aureus* or enterococci, in the absence of a primary focus *or* Microorganisms consistent with IE from persistently positive blood cultures defined as

— Two positive cultures of blood samples drawn >12 hours apart, or

— all of 3 or a majority of 4 separate cultures of blood (with first and last sample drawn 1 hour apart)

- *Evidence of endocardial involvement*

  Positive echocardiogram for IE defined as

  — oscillating intracardiac mass on valve or supporting structures, in the path of regurgitant jets, or on implanted material in the absence of an alternative anatomic explanation, or

  —new partial dehiscence of prosthetic valve

  — abscess

- New valvular regurgitation (worsening or changing of a preexisting murmur)

Minor criteria

- *Predisposition:* predisposing heart condition or intravenous drug abuse
- *Fever:* T> 38.0° C (100.4° F)
- *Vascular phenomena*: significant arterial emboli, septic pulmonary infarcts, mycotic aneurysm, intracranial hemorrhage, conjunctival hemorrhages, and Janeway lesions
- *Immunologic phenomena*: glomerulonephritis, Osler nodes, Roth spots, and rheumatoid factor
- *Microbiological evidence*: positive blood culture but does not meet a major criterion as noted below[1] or

serological evidence of active infection with organism consistent with IE

- *Echocardiographic findings*: compatible with IE but do not meet a major criterion as noted above

[1] Excludes single positive cultures for coagulase-negative staphylococci, diphtheroids, and organisms that do not commonly cause endocarditis.

MANAGEMENT

Overview

- resuscitation
- specific therapy: IV antibiotics +/- surgery
- supportive care and monitoring
- treat underlying cause and complications
- consults: infectious diseases, cardiology, cardiothoracic surgery

IV antibiotics

Empiric treatment for a community-acquired disease with a native valve:

- benzylpenicillin 1.8 g (child: 45 mg/kg (1.8 g max.) administration: IV, four times a day.
- Flucloxacillin 2 g (child: 50 mg/kg (2 g max.) IV, four times a day.

- gentamicin 4 to 6 mg/kg (child <10y: 7.5 mg/kg; 10y+: 6 mg/kg) IV, for 1st dose, then determine dosing interval for a maximum of either 1 or 2 further doses based on renal function)

- *Empirical treatment for hospital-acquired disease OR a prosthetic valve OR penicillin hypersensitivity OR suspected CA-MRSA:*
  vancomycin 1.5 g (child <12y: 30 mg/kg (1.5 g max.) IV, 12-hourly
  + gentamicin 4-6 mg/kg. (pediatric dose: <10y: 7.5 mg/kg; 10y+: 6 mg/kg) IV, for 1st dose, then calculate the dosing interval according to renal status)

- For low-risk patients, 1-2 weeks home-based therapy is sufficient.

- gentamicin is given q24h and is usually stopped after three doses unless proven streptococcal or enterococcal endocarditis (give q8h and continue)

- avoid clindamycin and lincomycin due to antibiotic resistance.

- directed therapy varies according to the main causative organism and the location valve affected

Surgery (valve replacement)

- indications

(1) hemodynamic instability
(2) abscess enlargement
(3) abscess (root, paravalvular, intracardiac)

(4) recurrent emboli
(5) organisms: *Staphylococcus aureus*, Q fever, fungal endocarditis

- early surgery (<48h) reduces long-term embolic complications, but usually, there is no effect on mortality.

PREVENTION

Overview

- there should be a more conservative approach as risks of adverse effects of antibiotics are more severe than threats of developing IE from surgical procedures.
- must have high-risk patient AND high-risk surgery

Risk assessment

- high-risk patients:

1. any prosthetic material used in valve repair
2. previous infectious endocarditis
3. congenital heart disease (unrepaired cyanotic, partially repaired, or if complete repair occurs in <6 months duration.)
4. Cardiac transplant patients with valvulopathy

- high-risk surgery

1. all dental procedures that involve procedures on gums or periapical region of teeth or perforation of the oral mucosa — thus only check-ups and simple fillings that don't involve gingiva don't need antibiotic prophylaxis

2. Respiratory tract surgery (procedures such as incision and biopsy, adenoidectomy, tonsillectomy)

Prophylactic Antibiotics:

a single dose of antibiotics should be given before the procedure or within 2 hours of the procedure

1. amoxicillin 50mg/kg PO
2. Cephazolin 50mg/kg IV/IM

For patients with Penicillin allergy:
1. clindamycin 20mg/kg PO (penicillin-allergic)

2. cephalexin 50mg/kg PO (penicillin-allergic)

COMPLICATIONS

- embolic (major arteries, brain, limbs, lungs, spleen, etc..)
- sepsis (local and metastatic abscess formation)
- valve incompetence and heart failure / cardiogenic shock
- arrhythmias
- death

Kawasaki Disease (Mucocutaneous Lymph Node Syndrome)

Kawasaki Disease (KD) is best described as a severe multi-system immune-mediated vasculitis of undetermined etiology.

- It is a disease of childhood and infancy as 85% of those affected are less than five years of age.
- KD is the most important cause of acquired heart disease in children in the US.
- The incidence of coronary artery aneurysm ranges from 15-25%iIn untreated patients of KD.
- Myocardial infarction, which occurs due to thrombotic occlusion of the coronary arteries, is the leading cause of death.
- This disease is more common in patients of Asian descent.
- Its prognosis depends on the magnitude of cardiac involvement and the swiftness in the start of medical treatment.

Pathogenesis

The etiology of KD is not known. In KD, the inflammation affects small to medium-sized arteries, including the coronary arteries. The first pathological change reported in the vessel wall is subendothelial collection of T-cells, mononuclear cells, macrophages, and monocytes.

The magnitude of coronary artery involvement is the critical factor that defines the extent of morbidity and mortality in a patient.

Clinical presentation

KD is distributed into three phases.

- The onset of high-grade fever in the absence of any focus marks the acute phase.

- Fever may last for 1-2 weeks.
- Acute myocardial infarction may develop during this phase due to vasculitis and perivasculitis.
- the fever recedes In the subacute phase, which may last for 2-4 weeks,
- In this phase, the Desquamation of the skin and coronary artery aneurysms appears.
- The platelet count increases and may increase above 106 per mm3.
- Acute phase reactants, for example, ESR and CRP, are usually raised.
- During the convalescent phase, usually within 6-8 weeks after onset of the illness, the symptoms are settled, and the platelet count and ESR return to normal.

Making the Diagnosis

Kawasaki Disease is a clinical diagnosis.

<u>The following criteria diagnose classic KD:</u>

Any four of the following criteria coupled with Fever of unknown origin lasting for at least five days

- Bilateral non-purulent conjunctivitis
- cracked and erythematous lips, strawberry tongue
- erythema of the hands and feet and desquamation of the skin on the fingers and toes
- maculopapular, erythema multiforme-like (or scarlatiniform) rash on extremities, trunk, and perineal regions

- One-sided Cervical lymphadenopathy (> 1.5 cm in diameter)

Alternative diagnostic criteria: Fever for at least five days plus two or three of the clinical features of coronary artery abnormalities on transthoracic echocardiography

Additional laboratory criteria (not required for diagnosis):

- Anemia
- Cerebrospinal fluid pleocytosis
- Elevated C-reactive protein and erythrocyte sedimentation rate
- Elevated liver enzyme levels
- Hypoalbuminemia < 3.0 g/dl
- Hyponatremia
- Platelets > 450 per mm3 after the first week
- Sterile pyuria
- White blood cell count > 15,000/uL

ECG findings:

- tachycardia,
- prolonged PR interval,
- ST-T wave changes,
- the decreased voltage of R waves may signify myocarditis.
- Q waves or ST-T wave changes may suggest MI.

Other investigations:

- Echo may show pericardial effusion, mitral insufficiency, LV dilation, and decreased systolic function.
- In the acute phase, Coronary angiography should not be done but may be needed later to evaluate the extent of coronary involvement.

Incomplete (Atypical Kawasaki Disease)

In a few cases, patients do not fulfill the standard criteria for Kawasaki disease and are categorized as having an incomplete (atypical) disease. Incomplete Kawasaki disease is more common in younger infants and older children.

Treatment of Acute Disease:

- A single IVIG (2 g/kg).
- High dose aspirin 80-100 mg/kg/day
- Corticosteroids
- Pentoxifylline "an inhibitor of TNF-alpha RNA transcription."
- varicella and influenza vaccine should be administered to children.
- After administration of a high dose of IVIG, Measles and varicella vaccines should be avoided for 11 months

Treatment of Refractory Disease:

- A second dose of 2 g/kg IVIG is recommended
- Pulse methylprednisolone

- Abciximab may be considered

Patients with moderate-sized aneurysms are treated with aspirin in combination with other antiplatelet agents such as clopidogrel (Plavix) or dipyridamole (Persantine).

For prevention and treatment of thrombosis, a combination of aspirin and LMWH or warfarin is used.

Cardiac catheterization is recommended for the patients presenting with clinical signs of angina or ischemic changes on a stress test.

3. Follow up of KD: serial echocardiograms should be done until Aneurysms subside entirely.

ECG after blunt cardiac trauma

Blunt cardiac injury (BCI) is best described as the injury suffered due to blunt trauma to the heart and chest. The symptoms of BCI range from clinically silent, transient arrhythmias to fatal cardiac wall rupture. The diagnosis of blunt cardiac injury is challenging due to the absence of a clear definition and a gold-standard test for laboratory workup. Treatment is customized to the severity of the injury and extends from EKG monitoring to sternotomy with complicated surgical repair. A high index of suspicion and monitoring is crucial for the early diagnosis of blunt cardiac trauma. Many patients are either asymptomatic or most commonly complain of chest pain, but this can be confused with the pain due to chest wall injuries. More significantly, BCI may express as a shock, which must be differentiated from other causes of hypotension such as neurogenic shock, tension pneumothorax, and hypovolemic shock.

In the case of BCI, EKGs are a useful screening tool and may detect rhythm and conduction disturbances. But it should be noted that there is no pathognomonic finding an EKG, which can help to make reliable diagnose of BCI.

PORTION 4:
ECG AND CARDIAC PACEMAKERS

CHAPTER 19:
ECG with cardiac pacemakers

A cardiac pacemaker is described as a medical device that generates electrical pulses. These impulses are delivered to heart muscles through specific electrodes. This device causes the heart muscle chambers to contract and therefore pump blood just like a natural pacemaker of the heart (SA-node).

Pacemaker Components

1. Pulse generator

- Power source
- Battery
- Control circuitry
- Transmitter / Receiver
- Reed Switch (Magnet triggered switch)

2. Lead(s)

- Single or multiple
- Unipolar or bipolar

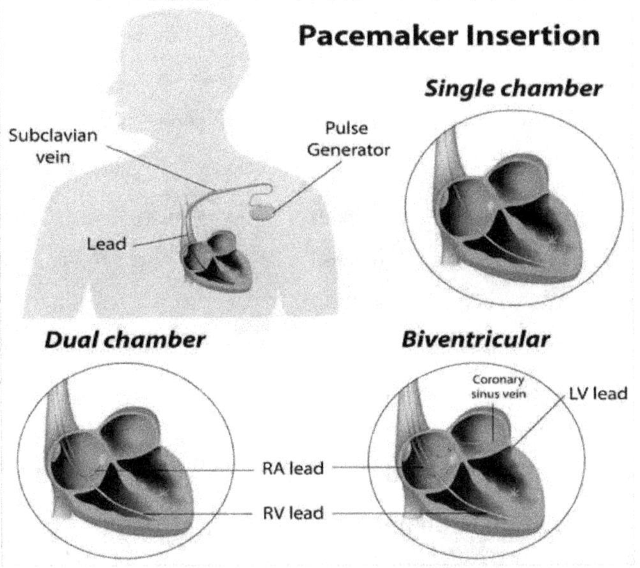

Pacemaker Classification

- The kind of their pacing mode classifies pacemakers.
- Classification follows pacemaker code is developed by the North American Society of Pacing and Electrophysiology (NASPE) and the British Pacing and Electrophysiology Group (BPEG).
- In 2002, The latest NASPE/BPEG Generic (NBG) Pacemaker Code was revised.
- The code is expressed as a sequence of up to five letters.

NBG Pacemaker Code (2002)

Position I	Position II	Position III	Position IV	Position V
Chamber(s)Paced	Chamber(s)Sensed	Response to Sensing	Rate Modulation	Multisite Pacing
O = None	O = None	O = None	O = None	O = None
A = Atrium	A = Atrium	T = Triggered	R = Rate Modulation	A = Atrium
V = ventricle	V = ventricle	I = Inhibited		V = ventricle
D = Dual (A+V)	D = Dual (A+V)	D = Dual (T+I)		D = Dual (A+V)

- **Position I:** Chambers Paced
  - Refers to chambers paced(atria or ventricle)
- **Position II:** Chambers Sensed
  - This refers to the location where the pacemaker senses natural cardiac electrical activity.
- **Position III:** Response to Sensing
  - This refers to the pacemaker's response to sensed natural cardiac activity.
  - T = Sensed activity results in generating of paced activity
  - I = Sensed activity results in decreasing of pacing activity
- **Position IV:** Rate Modulation
  - Indicates ability for a rate adjustment designed to altered heart suitably to meet

physiological needs, e.g., physical activity. Sensors may measure and respond to variable activities, including vibration, respiration, or acid-base status.

- **Position V:** Multisite Pacing
    - Allows indication of numerous stimulation sites within one anatomical area, e.g., more than one pacing location within the atria or biatrial pacing

Common Pacing Modes

AAI – Atrial pacing and sensing

- If natural atrial activity is sensed, then pacing is inhibited.
- If no native activity is sensed for a specific period, then atrial pacing initiated.
- Used in cases of sinus node dysfunction with intact AV conduction pathway
- Also termed as atrial demand mode.

VVI – Ventricle pacing and sensing

- Like AAI mode but involving ventricles instead of the atrium.
- They are used in patients with chronic atrial pathologies, e.g., atrial fibrillation or flutter.

DDD – pacing and sensing both the atria and ventricles

- Most common pacing mode.
- Atrial pacing occurs if no regular atrial activity is seen for a set time.
- Ventricular pacing occurs if no natural ventricle activity for a set time following atrial activity.
- Atrial channel function is suspended during a fixed period following atrial and ventricular activity to prevent sensing ventricular activity or retrograde p-waves as a regular activity.

Magnet mode

- Attaching a magnet to a pacemaker will initiate the magnet mode.
- This mode varies with pacemaker format and manufacturer.
- Generally initiates an asynchronous pacing mode – AOO, VOO, or DOO.
- Asynchronous modes deliver regularly paced stimuli at a constant rate regardless of natural rate or rhythm.
- In asynchronous ventricle pacing, there is a threat of pacemaker-induced ventricular tachycardia.
- The magnet used to an Implantable Cardioversion Defibrillator (ICD) results in defibrillator deactivation.

Criteria for Pacemaker Insertion:

- 2002--- American College of Cardiology, American Heart Association, and North American Society for Pacing and Electrophysiology guidelines for implantation of cardiac pacemakers.
- ACC/AHA/HRS --2008 Guidelines for Device-Based Therapy of Cardiac Rhythm Abnormalities

Paced ECG – Electrocardiographic Features

The appearance of the ECG in a patient with a cardiac pacemaker, dependents on the placement of pacing leads, pacing mode used, device pacing thresholds, and the presence of natural electrical activity. Features of the paced ECG are:

Pacing spikes

- Vertical spikes of short duration, generally of 2 ms.
- May not be visible in all leads.
- Amplitude depends on the location of the insertion and type of lead.
- Bipolar leads show a much smaller pacing spike than unipolar leads.
- Leads placed on epicardium produce in smaller pacing spikes than endocardial placed leads.

Atrial Pacing

- Pacing spike precedes the p wave.
- The shape of the p wave dependent upon lead placement but may appear normal.

Ventricular Pacing

- Pacing spike goes before the QRS complex.
- Right ventricle pacing leads placement results in a QRS morphology like LBBB.
- The Left epicardial pacing lead placement results in a QRS morphology the same as RBBB.
- ST segments and T waves are not in normal position with respect to the QRS complex, i.e., the terminal portion of the QRS complex is found on the opposite side of the baseline from the ST-segment and T-wave.

Dual-Chamber Pacing

- Dependent on areas being paced.
- May show characteristics of atrial pacing, ventricular pacing, or both.
- Pacing spikes may head before, only p wave, only QRS complex, or both.

The lack of paced complexes does not always mean pacemaker failure. It may indicate satisfactory native conduction.

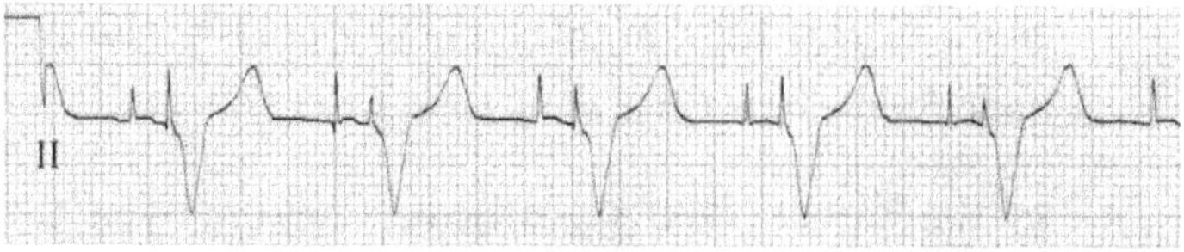

Atrial and ventricular pacing spikes

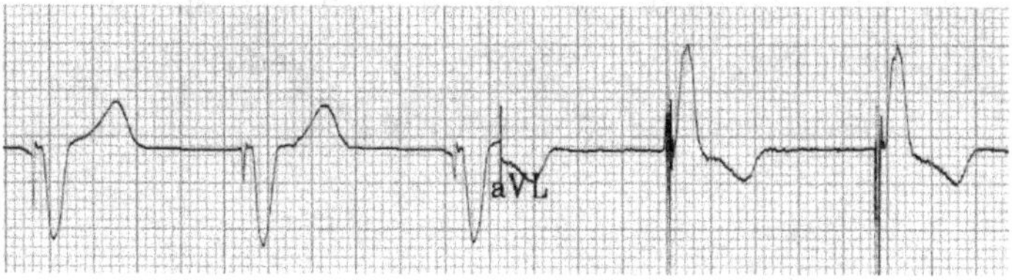

Regular discordance in a ventricular paced rhythm

ECG Examples

<u>Dual-Chamber Pacing:</u>

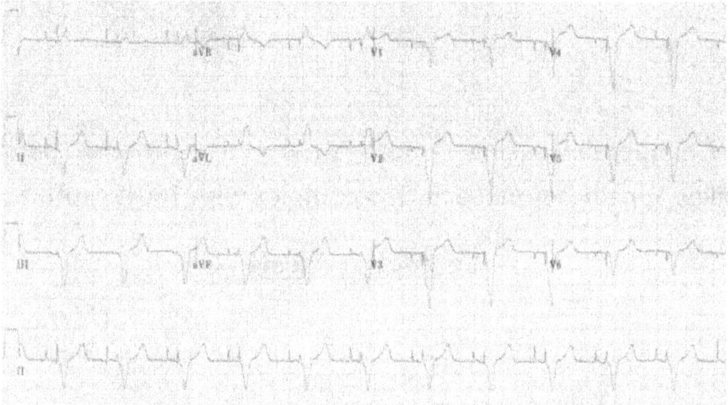

A-V sequential pacing:

- Both Atrial and ventricular pacing spikes are visible before each QRS complex.

- In the case of 100% atrial capture — small P waves are seen following each atrial pacing spike.
- In the case of 100% ventricular capture — a QRS complex follows each ventricular pacing spike.
- QRS complexes are broad with a shape of LBBB indicating the presence of a ventricular pacing electrode in the right ventricle.

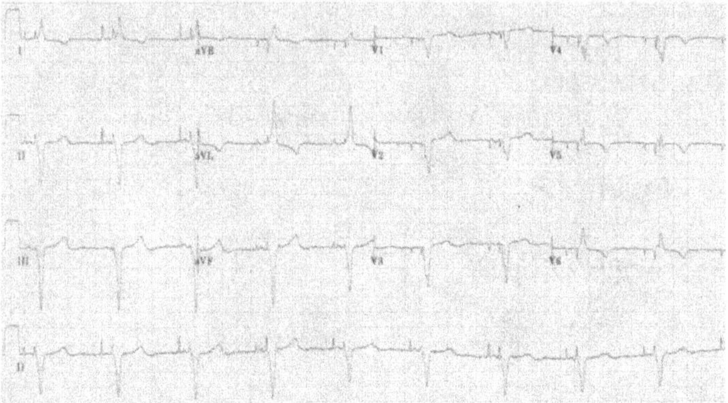

A-V sequential pacing -- both atrial and ventricular pacing spikes appear before each QRS complex with 100% capture.

<u>Ventricular Pacing</u>

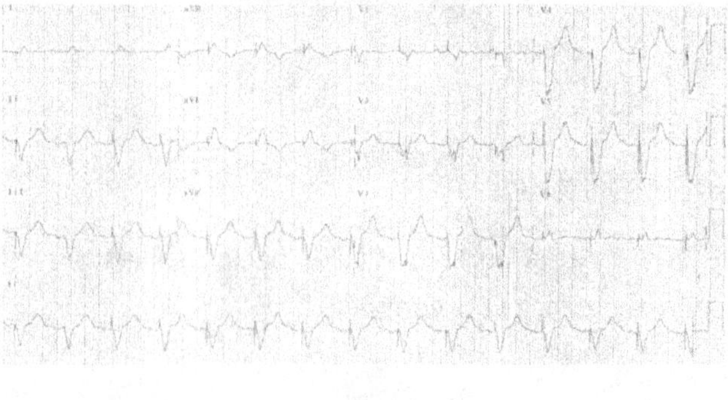

Ventricular paced rhythm:

- Ventricular pacing spikes precede each QRS complex
- No atrial pacing spikes are seen.
- The underlying natural rhythm is probably coarse atrial fibrillation — there are several possible P waves visible in V1

Capture beats:

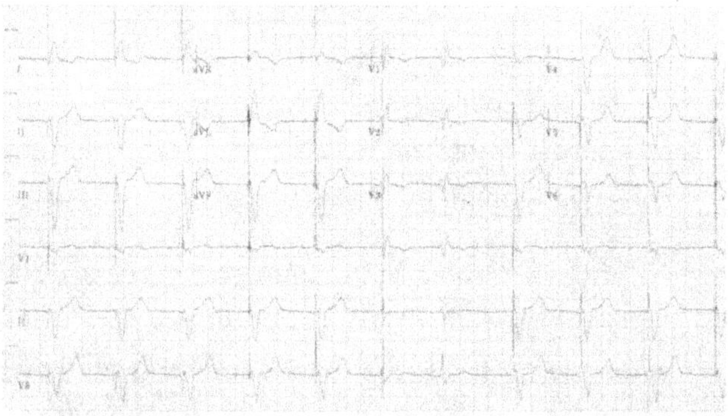

- most of the QRS complexes follow the Ventricular pacing spikes.
- In the above ECG, The 6th and 7th beats are narrower, with a different morphology— these are non-paced ("capture") beats

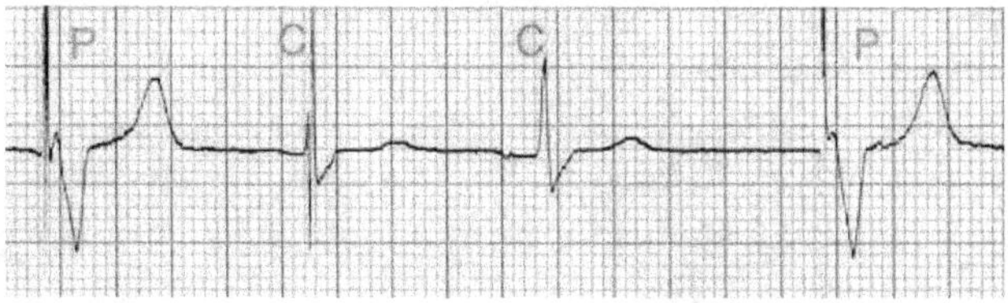

P = paced beat, C = capture beat

Fusion beats:

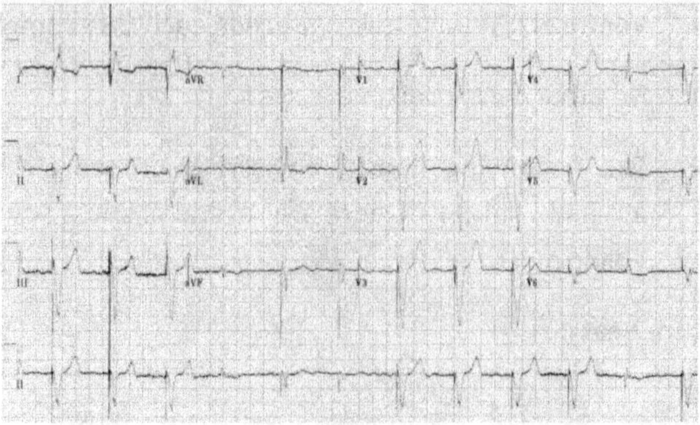

- Ventricular pacing spikes appear before the QRS complexes, most of which show LBBB morphology coherent with an RV pacing electrode.
- The 5th, 6th, and 11th complexes have a different morphology— these are **fusion beats.** It is produced when the ventricle is simultaneously activated by both paced and supraventricular (natural) impulses. The pacing spike is short, and the co-incident natural impulse narrows the QRS duration.

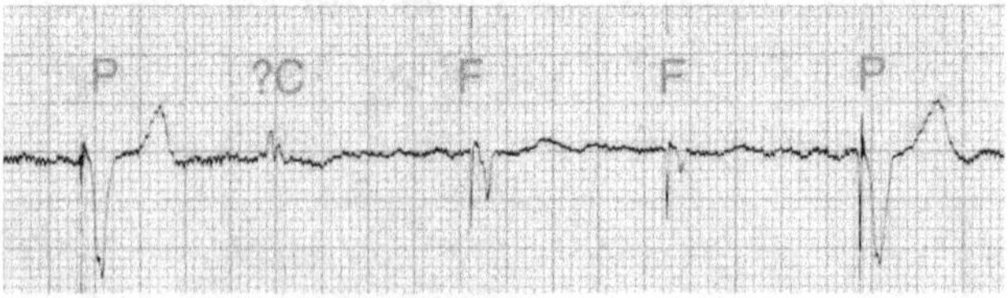

In the ECG above P stands for the paced beat, F stands for fusion beat, and C stands for capture beat

Atrial Pacing

Patients with atrial placed cardiac pacemakers often show 1st degree AV block or Wenckebach conduction on their paced ECG, which was not apparent on their baseline tracing.

This is because when these patients are paced at a rate faster than their AV node can handle, as the AV node eventually becomes "fatigued or exhausted," 1st degree AV block occurs known as Wenckebach phenomenon on the paced ECG. This abnormality is not clinically significant, provided that the patient's cardiac output is not compromised.

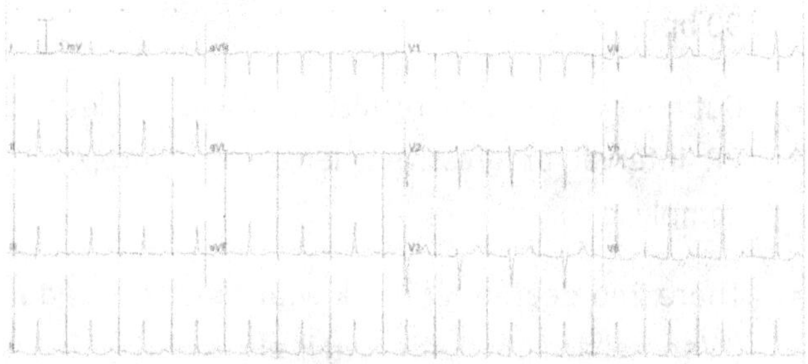

In the ECG above Atrial paced rhythm with 1st degree AV block is shown

- There are regularly pacing spikes at 90 bpm.
- P wave precedes Each pacing spike (100% atrial capture)
- with a prolonged PR interval (280 ms) P waves are conducted to the ventricles.

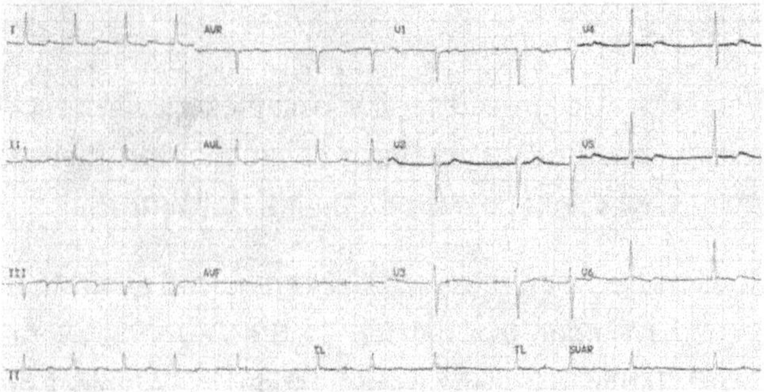

In the above ECG tracing Atrial paced rhythm with Wenckebach conduction is shown

- A small P wave follows regular atrial pacing spikes at 90 bpm
- But not every P wave results in a QRS complex and the PR interval progressively lengthens ("dropped QRS complexes").
- There 2nd degree AV block with Mobitz I conduction (Wenckebach phenomenon) is also seen.

CHAPTER 20:
Pacemaker Malfunctioning and ECG

Pacemaker malfunction can occur for a variety of reasons, varying from equipment failure to changes in an underlying natural rhythm.

Diagnosis of pacemaker malfunction is very challenging and often associated with non-specific clinical symptoms. On the other hand, ECG changes can be delicate or absent.

Problems with Sensing

Under-sensing

- This occurs when the pacemaker fails to sense natural cardiac activity.
- This Results in asynchronous pacing.
- Causes include an increased threshold for the stimulus at the electrode site (exit block), poor contact of lead with the target tissue, new bundle branch block, or problems in programming.
- ECG findings may be minimal, even though the presence of pacing spikes within QRS complexes is suggestive of understanding.

Oversensing

- Oversensing occurs when electrical signals are inappropriately recognized as natural cardiac activity and pacing is inhibited.
- These improper signals may be in the form of large P or T waves, skeletal muscle activity, or lead contact problems.
- Abnormal signals may not be apparent on ECG.
- Reduced pacemaker output or output failure may be seen on ECG monitoring if the patient increases their rectus or pectoral muscle movements (due to oversensing of muscle activity).

Problems with Pacing

Output failure

- when a paced stimulus is not generated according to the body requirement, it is known as Output failure.
- This results in decreased or absent pacemaker function.
- Many other causes, including oversensing, wire damage, lead displacement, or interference.

Failure to capture

- Failure to capture often occurs when the paced stimulus does not result in myocardial depolarization.

- Other causes including electrode displacement, wire damage, electrolyte disturbance, Myocardial ischemia, or exit block.

If the patient's natural heart rate is above the pacemaker limit, no pacemaker activity should be expected, and therefore on ECG, output failure and capture failure will be recognized.

Pacemaker Associated Dysrhythmias

Several types of pacemaker associated dysrhythmias can happen including

- pacemaker-mediated tachycardia (PMT)
- sensor-induced tachycardia
- runaway pacemaker
- pacemaker-mediated Wenckebach AV block
- lead dislodgement dysrhythmia.

Pacemaker-mediated tachycardia (PMT)

- Its other names are endless-loop tachycardia or pacemaker circus movement tachycardia.

- PMT is described as a re-entry tachycardia in which the pacemaker forms the antegrade path, and AV node creates a retrograde path for backward signal transmission.

- Cretrograde p waves being sensed as a natural atrial activity with succeeding ventricular pacing.

- The paced ventricular complex results in additional backward conduction of signals with the generation of retrograde p wave, thus forming a continuous cycle.
- This results in a paced tachycardia with the maximum rate controlled by the pacemaker programming.
- It can be dismissed by slowing AV conduction, e.g., adenosine or activation of magnet mode.
- The new generation of pacemakers contains programmed algorithms designed to terminate PMT.
- May ensue rate-related ischemia in the presences of Ischemic heart disease.

Sensor-induced tachycardia

- In response to physiological stimuli, modern pacemakers are programmed to adjust heart rate accordingly, e.g., maintain heart rate after exercise and in case of fever.
- Sensors may "misfire" in the presence of disturbing stimuli such as vibrations, loud noises, fever, limb movement, hyperventilation, or electrocautery (for instance, during surgery).
- This misfiring leads to pacing at an improperly fast rate.
- The ventricular rate did not exceed the pacemaker's upper rate limit (usually 160-180 bpm).

- These will also normally terminate with the application of a magnet.

Runaway pacemaker

- This potentially lethal malfunction of older-generation pacemakers is related to low battery voltage (e.g., overdue pacemaker replacement).
- The pacemaker delivers outbursts of pacing spikes at 2000 bpm, which may provoke ventricular fibrillation.
- Surprisingly, there may be a failure to capture, resulting in bradycardia. It occurs when the pacing spikes are very low in amplitude (due to the depleted battery voltage).
- By applying magnet in case of emergency can be lifesaving, but definitive treatment requires replacement of the pacemaker.

Lead displacement dysrhythmia

- A misplaced pacing lead may drift around inside the right ventricle, occasionally irritating the myocardium and causing ventricular ectopics or runs of VT, alternating with failure of capture.
- If the paced QRS shape changes from an LBBB pattern (indicating RV placement) to an RBBB pattern (indicating LV placement), this indicates that the electrode has worn through the interventricular septum.

- A chest x-ray will generally help to confirm the diagnosis.

Pacemaker Syndrome

- It is caused by improper timing of atrial and ventricular contractions resulting in AV improper synchrony and loss of atrial "kick."
- Range of clinical symptoms, includes fatigue, dizziness, palpations, pre-syncope.
- There is an associated decrease in systolic blood pressure > 20 mmHg during the change from natural rhythm to a paced rhythm.

Twiddler's Syndrome

- The patient manipulates the pulse generator (accidentally or intentionally).
- If the pacemaker rotates on its long axis, this results in dislodgement of pacing leads.
- It can result in diaphragmatic or brachial plexus pacing (e.g., arms twitching) depending on the degree of lead migration.

ECG in Pacemaker Malfunction

- Normal pacemaker's malfunctions can result in absent pacing activity, irregular pacing, and absence of pacing spikes.

- Depending on the underlying natural rhythm, diagnosis of pacemaker malfunction on the ECG is challenging and maybe impossible.
- If pacemaker malfunction is speculated, cardiology review is necessary to assist in pacemaker interrogation and testing.

Example- Pacing failure:

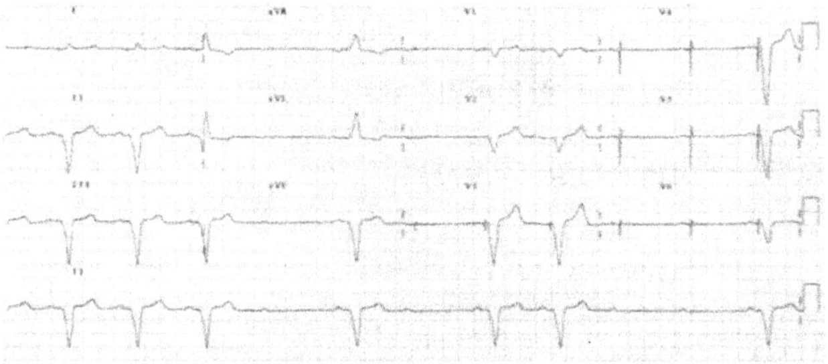

This ECG shows random **failure to capture beats** and a ventricular paced rhythm. Atrial sensing appears to be intact, and ventricular pacing spikes follow each P wave, most clearly seen in leads V3-6

Example- Rapid ventricular pacing

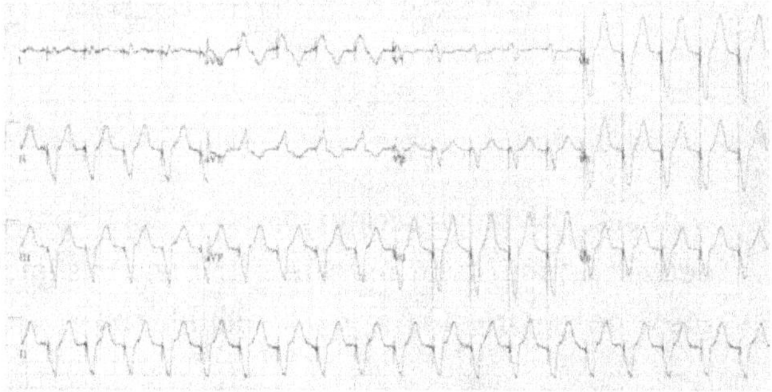

There is no evidence of preceding atrial activity, and there is a rapid ventricular-paced rhythm (120 bpm). The differential diagnosis of this rhythm would consist of:

- Pacemaker-mediated tachycardia in which there is a retrograde P wave buried in the QRS complexes /T waves.
- Sensor-induced tachycardia.
- It could potentially be normal in the presence of a proper physical stimulus (e.g., exercise).

Example – Runaway pacemaker

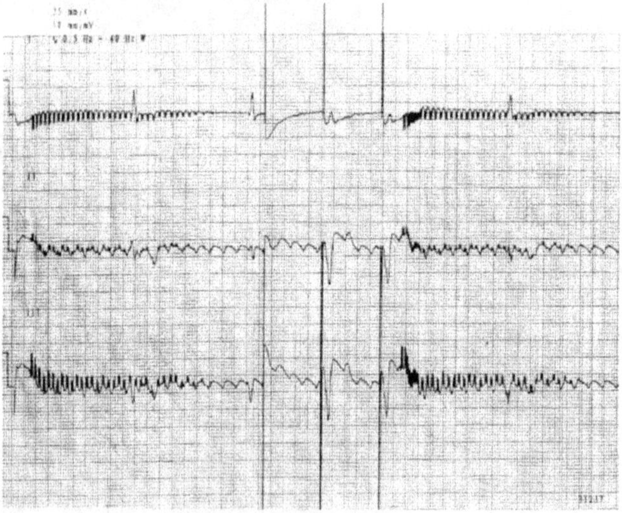

- Outbursts of rapid pacing spikes at 2000 bpm with decreasing amplitude and rate — this fails to stimulate the ventricles due to the low amplitude spikes.

- The main rhythm is of atrial flutter with 3rd degree AV block and ventricular escape rhythm at 30 bpm.
- three pacing spikes are seen In the middle

Some Quick Tips

1. on ECG, a left bundle branch block (LBBB) will be formed If a lead is in the right ventricle.
2. If the lead is in the LV, it will generate a right bundle branch block (RBBB) pattern. (Most permanent pacemakers seen in the emergency will have leads in the RV and have an LBBB pattern)
3. Paced spikes are not always noticeable in every lead.
4. Observe for unique beats:
    - ***Fusion beats*** – an odd hybrid of QRS complex forms when the native beat and pacemaker beat combine
    - ***Capture beats*** – the natural beat breaks through and is conducted by the ventricle. It is narrower and has a different shape than paced beats.

PORTION 5:

HISTORY OF ELECTROCARDIOGRA PHY AT A GLANCE

The word ECG derives from the German language. In German, it is elektro-kardiographie as it monitors the cardiac activity of the heart.

- **1775**--Abildgaard shows that hens became unconscious with electrical stimuli and he could reestablish a pulse with electrical shocks across the chest.
- **1786** – Italian Anatomist Luigi Galvani observed that a dissected frog's leg twitches when touched with a metal scalpel.
- **1788**--Charles Kite wrote an essay on the use of electricity in the diagnosis and resuscitation of a dead person.
- **1819**-- Danish physicist Hans Christian discovered electromagnetism
- **1827**--Leopoldo Nobili, managed to detect the flow of current in the body of a frog from muscles to the spinal cord.
- **1838**-- Carlo Matteucci, shows that an electric current accompanies each heartbeat.
- **1843**-- German physiologist Emil Du Bois-Reymond describes "action potential" associated with each muscular contraction.
- **1856**--Rudolph von Koelliker and Heinrich Muller prove that an electrical current comes with each heartbeat by applying a galvanometer to the dissected ventricle of the heart (at the apex and base of heart)

- **1858--**William Thompson invents the 'mirror galvanometer' for the reception of transatlantic telegraph transmissions.
- **1867--**Thompson improves telegraph transmissions with the 'Siphon Recorder' which could not only detect currents it could also record them onto paper.
- **1869-70**--Alexander Muirhead may have recorded a human electrocardiogram by using a Thompson Siphon Recorder, but he never published his work.
- **1873** – Gabriel Lippmann invented The capillary electrometer.
- **1873** – Luigi Luciani (1840 – 1919) explained about cardiac group beating (which he called periodic rhythm) and documented 2nd degree AV blocks while studying frogs hearts
- **1873** – Alfred Lewis Galabin (1843 – 1913) was the first scientist who demonstrated atrioventricular block in humans
- **1882**--John Burdon-Sanderson, was the first to coin the term "isoelectric interval."
- **1887--** Augustus Waller invented the ECG machine consisting of a Lippmann capillary electrometer fixed to a projector. It was the first ECG from the intact human heart.
- **1893** – Dutch physician and physiologist Willem Einthoven (1860 – 1927) introduces the term 'electro-cardiogramme

- **1895**--Willem Einthoven assigned the letters P, Q, R, S, and T to the deflections in the theoretical waveform.Einthoven also described the electrocardiographic characteristics of several cardiovascular disorders.
- **1897**--the string galvanometer was devised by the French engineer Clément Ader.
- **1901** –Einthoven invented Saitengalvanometer (string galvanometer).
- **1902** –Einthoven published the first ECG.
- **1905** – Einthoven delivers the first systematized presentation of normal and abnormal electrocardiograms recorded with his string galvanometer and recording apparatus in his laboratory.
- **1912**--Einthoven summarized his diagram of the equilateral triangle formed by his standard leads I, II and III (Einthoven triangle)
- **1924**-- Einthoven was awarded the Nobel Prize in Medicine for his pioneering work in developing the ECG.
- **1927**--General Electric had developed a handy machine that could produce electrocardiograms without the use of the string galvanometer.
- **1937**--Taro Takemi invented the new portable electrocardiograph machine.

- **1947** – Claude Schaeffer Beck (1894-1971) defibrillated a human heart successfully.
- **1953** – John J Osborn (1917 – 2014) studied the effect of hypothermia on the respiratory and cardiac function in dogs.provided information about j point on ECG and Osborn waves.
- **1957** –Anton Jervell (1901-1987) with his colleague and jazz virtuoso Fred Lange-Nielsen (1919-1989) explain about an autosomal recessive syndrome of long-QT interval
- **1963** – in 1963, Cesarino Romano (1924 – 2008) and In 196 4Owen Conor Ward, independently report an autosomal dominant variant of long QT syndrome (LQTS)that was *without* congenital hearing loss.
- **1966** – François Dessertenne described the first case of 'torsades de pointes.'
- **1967** – Professor Frank Pantridge (1916-2004) was the inventor of the first Western portable defibrillator (1965) and also published a report about the first pre-hospital resuscitation using the mobile coronary care unit (MCCU)
- **1967** – The "Minnesota code" for ECG classification was formed.
- **1976** – Erhardt, Sjögren, and Wahlberg explained the use of a right-sided precordial lead (CR_4R or V_4R) in the diagnosis of right ventricular infarction

- **1970** – Uhley HN wrote an article with the title of "Electrocardiographic telemetry from ambulances. A practical approach to mobile coronary care units. "

- **1977** – The epsilon waves are observed in 30% of patients with arrhythmogenic right ventricular dysplasia. It was the first time defined and described by Guy Fontaine (1936-2018).

- **1978** – Alois Langer, Marlin Heilman, Morton Mower, and Mieczyslaw Mirowski patented a device which they named as a "Circuit for monitoring a heart and for effecting cardioversion of a needy heart" This was the start of the era of the implantable cardiac defibrillator.

- **1996** – Elena B. Sgarbossa develops and supports a **Sgarbossa prediction** rule It was based on a set of ECG criteria for the diagnosis of acute myocardial infarction in patients with chest pain and left bundle-branch block

- **2005** – the 15-lead ECG, for assessing the diagnostic value of an ECG containing leads V4R, V8, and V9:

- **2008** – in 2008, The de Winter ECG pattern was first described as a case series by de Winter RJ

- **2018** – Apple smartwatch used to determine whether a wearable technology can identify irregular heart rhythms suggestive of atrial fibrillation.

- **2018** – Smartphone 12-lead ECG

NEW MODALITIES IN ECG:

Electrocardiogram (ECG) has been used as a necessary cardiac diagnostic tool for a century, and while the principle remains the same, testing systems are evolving to meet today's demands of new and better technology. This includes enhanced mobility, ease of use, streamlined workflow, and interoperability so data can be easily updated with electronic medical records.

ECG Automation for Diagnosis :

ECG interpretation algorithms now come on many systems. Gender- and age-specific criteria are used to provide a virtual second opinion for ECG interpretation.

Some systems have anatomical interfaces to help to reduce the chances of improper lead placement or recognition for the presence of a pacemaker.

ECG Workflow Improvements:

ECG systems have been made accessible to improve workflow. Examples include simplified step-by-step operation, electronic medical records (EMRs), the introduction of touch-screen, better connectivity with ECG management systems, and cardiovascular information systems (CVIS).

Need to Standardize ECG Formats:

The aim of healthcare reform IT requirements is to advance workflow, ease the transfer of patient data electronically and to eliminate the need for paper-based systems, including paper ECG waveforms.

Remote Access to ECGs

One advantage of paperless ECG is to review an electronic web-based ECG management system and to access ECGs outside of the traditional workstation and hospital settings. Thus enabling physicians for distant viewing and reporting.

Wearable and Remote ECG Monitoring:

The traditional 12-lead ECG system is a backbone in cardiac diagnostics in the clinical or hospital setting. But the future of cardiac assessment may shift to the evaluation by patients themselves before requiring analysis by physicians or other systems. There is now a tendency in Holter monitoring through inexpensive wearable or smartphone-based ECG monitors. With the elimination of electrode wires, these devices are more comfortable and handy now. These devices are either fixed on the patient's chest or connect with patients' cell phones to eliminate the need for an external hardwired in the patient's home.

CONCLUSION

There is an old story about a man and a start fish.

While going down the beach, a man saw someone in the distance leaning down, picking up something and tossing it in the ocean. As he came close by, he saw thousands of starfish the tide had thrown onto the beach. Unable to return to the sea during low tide, the starfish were dying. He found a young boy picking up the starfish one by one and throwing them back into the ocean. After watching the seemingly pointless effort, the man said, "There must be numerous starfish on this beach. It would be hard for you to save all of them. There are simply too many. You can't possibly save sufficient enough to make a difference." The young boy grinned as he picked up another starfish and threw it back into the sea and replied. "It has made a difference to that one,"

The medical field is as vast and deep, just like an ocean. There are millions of clinical facts, and figures and NO body can remember these all. Similarly, in one's clinical career, he will meet several patients, but one can't save them all.

But just by acquiring enough and precise medical knowledge, one can make a significant difference in someone's life. Learning how to interpret ECG is one of those lifesaving skills.

ECG, since its time of invention, has made a substantial change in the field of medicine. It is now taken as one of the baseline investigations for the diagnosis of conditions related to the heart. It is non-invasive and easily accessible. It is one of the essential tests for evaluating the abnormalities associated with cardiac rhythm. Timely detection of myocardial ischemia and myocardial infarction is only made possible due to ECG. Defects in the conduction system, preexcitation, long QT syndromes, atrial anomalies, ventricular hypertrophy, pericarditis, are few of other disorders which can be diagnosed by ECG.

Cardiovascular disease is considered the number one cause of death. It puts a great emphasis on health-care providers to develop skills and knowledge in interpreting ECGs to provide the best care promptly. Many health-care providers find the advanced interpretation of ECG findings a complicated task. Errors in the analysis can lead to misdiagnosis resulting in delaying the appropriate treatment.

This book is a little effort to make this difficult task simple, but the only way to master the ECG is to do repeated ECG interpretation exercises.

CPSIA information can be obtained
at www.ICGtesting.com
Printed in the USA
BVHW081142261020
591816BV00001B/169